Quick Questions in
Heat-Related Illness and Hydration

Expert Advice in Sports Medicine

QUICK QUESTIONS IN SPORTS MEDICINE

SERIES

SERIES EDITOR, ERIC L. SAUERS, PHD, ATC, FNATA

Quick Questions in
Heat-Related Illness and Hydration
Expert Advice in Sports Medicine

Editor

Rebecca M. Lopez, PhD, ATC, CSCS
Assistant Professor
Department of Orthopaedics and Sports Medicine
Morsani College of Medicine
University of South Florida
Tampa, Florida

Series Editor

Eric L. Sauers, PhD, ATC, FNATA
Professor and Chair
Department of Interdisciplinary Health Sciences
Arizona School of Health Sciences
A.T. Still University
Mesa, Arizona

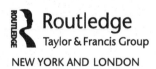
Routledge
Taylor & Francis Group

NEW YORK AND LONDON

First published in 2015 by National Athletic Trainers' Association & SLACK Incorporated

Published 2024 by Routledge
605 Third Avenue, New York, NY 10158

and by Routledge
4 Park Square, Milton Park, Abingdon, Oxon OX14 4RN

Routledge is an imprint of the Taylor & Francis Group, an informa business

The "Quick Questions in Heat-Related Illness and Hydration: Expert Advice in Sports Medicine" book ("Heat-Related Illness and Hydration Book") is © 2015 by National Athletic Trainers' Association and Taylor & Francis Group.

Library of Congress Cataloging-in-Publication Data

Quick questions in heat-related illness and hydration : expert advice in sports medicine / editor, Rebecca M. Lopez.
   p. ; cm.
Includes bibliographical references and index.
ISBN 978-1-61711-647-6 (alk. paper)
I. Lopez, Rebecca M., 1976- , editor.
  [DNLM: 1. Athletic Performance--physiology. 2. Heat Stress Disorders. 3. Athletic Injuries--metabolism. 4. Dehydration--physiopathology. 5. Sports--physiology. 6. Sports Medicine--methods. WD 610]
  RC963.5.H4
  616.9'89--dc23
                         2014047741

ISBN: 9781617116476 (pbk)
ISBN: 9781003526124 (ebk)

DOI: 10.4324/9781003526124

DEDICATION

This book is dedicated to the individuals who have lost their lives to exertional heat stroke or other causes of sudden death in sport, and to the athletic trainers and other health care providers caring for the physically active.

Contents

ACKNOWLEDGMENTS

There is no way I could have completed this project on my own. There are several people I would like to thank for their efforts and support throughout the development of this book.

To my contributing authors: Thank you for all of your efforts. I truly enjoyed working with each and every one of you on this project, and I am glad to have you as my colleagues.

Thank you to Dr. Doug Casa, Dr. Becca Stearns, and the rest of the crew from the Korey Stringer Institute. We share the same passion and drive to make things better. This book would not have been possible without you.

To my USF colleagues and students: A special thanks to Steve and Amanda for being my sounding board, as well as to the athletic training students who assisted and modeled for some of the photos.

Thank you to the series editor, Dr. Eric Sauers, and to SLACK Incorporated, for the opportunity to be a part of this book series and for your support throughout the process. Thank you to Brien Cummings for always having an answer to my many questions.

Thank you to my mom, sister, and the rest of my family and friends for their constant love and support. Last, a special thanks to Betty for her aesthetic vision, motivation, moral support, and love, now and always.

ABOUT THE EDITOR

Rebecca M. Lopez, PhD, ATC, CSCS graduated from Florida International University in 1998 with a Bachelor's of Science in Health Education, Athletic Training Specialization. She returned to Florida International University and obtained her Master of Science in Advanced Athletic Training/Sports Medicine in 2004. She completed her PhD in Kinesiology from the University of Connecticut in 2010. Dr. Lopez is a Board-Certified Athletic Trainer, an American College of Sports Medicine Certified Health Fitness Specialist, and a Certified Strength and Conditioning Specialist through the National Strength and Conditioning Association. She worked as a certified athletic trainer in Miami-Dade Public Schools for several years and has volunteered in the medical tent at the Boston Marathon, Marine Corps Marathon, Falmouth Road Race, and others. Her research interests include exertional heat stroke and other exertional heat illnesses, cooling methods for hyperthermic athletes, ergogenic aids and thermoregulation, sickle cell trait in athletes, hydration and exercise performance, and preventing sudden death in sports. She has published numerous peer-reviewed articles and several chapters on exertional heat illness, hydration, and preventing sudden death in sports. Dr. Lopez is currently an Assistant Professor in the Department of Orthopaedics and Sports Medicine and the Director of the Post-Professional Graduate Athletic Training Program at the University of South Florida. She also serves on the medical and science advisory board for the Korey Stringer Institute.

CONTRIBUTING AUTHORS

J. D. Adams, MS (Question 36)
Research Assistant
Human Performance Laboratory
University of Arkansas
Fayetteville, Arkansas

William M. Adams, MS, ATC
(Questions 15, 20)
Korey Stringer Institute
University of Connecticut
Storrs, Connecticut

Candi D. Ashley, PhD (Questions 12, 38)
University of South Florida
Tampa, Florida

Joseph S. Atkin, MD (Question 17)
Fellow
Orthopaedics and Sports Medicine
University of South Florida
Tampa, Florida

Luke N. Belval, ATC, CSCS
(Questions 14, 19)
Director of Special Projects
Korey Stringer Institute
University of Connecticut
Storrs, Connecticut

Michele C. Benz, MS, ATC, CSCS (Question 5)
Head Athletic Trainer
Miami Palmetto Senior High
Miami-Dade County Public Schools
Miami, Florida

Douglas J. Casa, PhD, ATC, FACSM, FNATA
(Questions 1, 11, 19)
Korey Stringer Institute
Department of Kinesiology
University of Connecticut
Storrs, Connecticut

Michelle A. Cleary, PhD, ATC
(Questions 4, 8, 28)
Associate Professor of Athletic Training
Crean College of Health and
   Behavioral Science
Chapman University
Orange, California

Earl R. "Bud" Cooper, EdD, ATC, CSCS
(Question 25)
Associate Clinical Professor
The University of Georgia
Athens, Georgia

Eric E. Coris, MD (Question 17)
Professor
Department of Family Medicine
Department of Orthopedics and
   Sports Medicine
Morsani College of Medicine
University of South Florida
Tampa, Florida

Julie K. DeMartini, PhD, ATC
(Questions 13, 21, 22)
Assistant Professor/Athletic Training
   Program Director
Westfield State University
Westfield, Massachusetts

Deanna M. Dempsey, MS (Questions 6, 32)
Assistant Director of Elite Athlete
   Health and Performance
Korey Stringer Institute
University of Connecticut
Storrs, Connecticut

Lindsey E. Eberman, PhD, LAT, ATC
  (Questions 23, 29)
Post-Professional Athletic Training
Program Director
Associate Professor
Department of Applied Medicine and
  Rehabilitation
College of Nursing, Health, and
  Human Services
Indiana State University
Terre Haute, Indiana

Dawn M. Emerson, MS, ATC
  (Questions 34, 35)
University of South Carolina
Columbia, South Carolina

Matthew S. Ganio, PhD (Questions 3, 30, 37)
Director
Human Performance Laboratory
Department of Health, Human
  Performance and Recreation
University of Arkansas
Fayetteville, Arkansas

Yuri Hosokawa, MAT, ATC, LAT (Question 11)
Korey Stringer Institute
University of Connecticut
Storrs, Connecticut

Robert A. Huggins, PhD, ATC, LAT
  (Questions 21, 26)
Director of Elite Athlete Health and
  Performance
Korey Stringer Institute
University of Connecticut
Storrs, Connecticut

Evan C. Johnson, PhD (Question 39)
Department of Health, Human
  Performance, and Recreation
University of Arkansas
Fayetteville, Arkansas

Stavros A. Kavouras, PhD, FACSM, FECSS
  (Questions 36, 39)
Associate Professor
Coordinator
Exercise Science Program
Human Performance Laboratory
University of Arkansas
Fayetteville, Arkansas

Brendon P. McDermott, PhD, ATC
  (Questions 27, 31)
Assistant Professor/Clinical Coordinator
Graduate Athletic Training
  Education Program
Department of Health, Human
  Performance and Recreation
University of Arkansas
Fayetteville, Arkansas

Nicole E. Moyen, MS, CSCS (Question 30)
Human Performance Laboratory
Department of Health, Human
  Performance, and Recreation
University of Arkansas
Fayetteville, Arkansas

Francis G. O'Connor, MD, MPH
  (Questions 16, 26)
Professor and Chair
Military and Emergency Medicine
Associate Director
Consortium for Health and
  Military Performance (CHAMP)
Uniformed Services University of the
  Health Sciences
Bethesda, Maryland

Robert C. Oh, MD, MPH (Question 16)
Sports Medicine
Department of Family Medicine
Uniformed Services University of the
  Health Sciences
Bethesda, Maryland

Nicholas D. Peterkin, MD (Question 17)
Sports and Family Medicine
Baptist Primary Care
Jacksonville, Florida

J. Luke Pryor, MS, ATC, CSCS
(Questions 9, 18, 32)
Department of Kinesiology
University of Connecticut
Storrs, Connecticut

Riana R. Pryor, MS, ATC
(Questions 1, 9, 18, 20)
Korey Stringer Institute
Department of Kinesiology
University of Connecticut
Storrs, Connecticut

Mike D. Ryan, PT, ATC, CES, PES
(Question 33)
Mike Ryan Sports Medicine, Inc
Jacksonville Beach, Florida

Rebecca L. Stearns, PhD, ATC
(Questions 6, 7, 13, 24)
Korey Stringer Institute
University of Connecticut
Storrs, Connecticut

Matthew A. Tucker, MA (Question 37)
Human Performance Laboratory
Department of Health, Human
    Performance, and Recreation
University of Arkansas
Fayetteville, Arkansas

Lesley W. Vandermark, MS, ATC, PES
(Questions 14, 15)
Korey Stringer Institute
University of Connecticut
Storrs, Connecticut

PREFACE

The Quick Questions series was developed to provide clinicians with brief, direct, actionable answers to clinical questions that they encounter in the daily practice of sports medicine to help optimize patient care. Today, information access is easier than it has ever been. However, it is a challenge to find the time and develop the skill to consume and synthesize large bodies of evidence to distill knowledge into action. Because we typically do not have the time to complete this daunting task for every clinical question that arises, we often turn to our peers and colleagues for advice. One of the most trusted sources of information in health care is the expert consult. The Quick Questions series is like having a team of sports medicine experts with you on the sidelines to provide you with concise, straightforward advice to answer your most important clinical questions.

The editor of each book is a leading expert in his or her area of sports medicine practice who has assembled a team of expert clinicians and scholars to develop answers to 39 of the most commonly posed and clinically important questions. Each book is a compendium of expert advice from clinicians with the knowledge and experience to help guide your clinical decision making to provide safe and effective patient care.

In this book, *Quick Questions in Heat-Related Illness and Hydration: Expert Advice in Sports Medicine*, Dr. Rebecca M. Lopez and her team of expert contributing authors have answered 39 of the most important clinical questions regarding some of the most preventable, yet life-threatening, issues in sports medicine. This book begins with an appropriately strong emphasis on prevention of heat-related illnesses. Next, the focus turns to the diagnosis and emergency management of heat-related illness. Subsequently, a section on special considerations, including environmental conditions and return to play, addresses key areas that can pose challenges for clinicians. The final section of the book focuses on hydration and includes answers to a wide variety of questions regarding topics such as fluid intake, hyponatremia, measuring hydration status, and the effects of sodium.

With the busy schedules, job stresses, and time constraints inherent to sports medicine practice, it is my sincere hope that this series proves to be a valuable resource full of expert advice that you find helpful in caring for your patients and athletes.

Eric L. Sauers, PhD, ATC, FNATA
Series Editor

Introduction

Similar to other topics in athletic training, some of the information pertaining to exertional heat illnesses and hydration in older athletic training textbooks and other sources of information were based on anecdotal reports from the field. However, research in this area has made significant progress in the past few decades. As such, the evidence-based research and information available to athletic trainers and other health care professionals has been extremely beneficial to clinicians and the patients they care for. With my clinical experiences at the high school level in South Florida for nearly 10 years, I grew to understand what it was like to care for hundreds of athletes in a hot, humid environment. Looking back, the combination of the environment, a few difficult coaches, unacclimatized and unfit athletes, and a "this is how we learned back in the day" mentality for treating heat illnesses may have been dangerous. As I entered the world of research while still practicing clinically, I began to realize how far we were as a profession in providing the best clinical care when it came to hydration and heat illnesses. I was enthralled with the idea of merging those 2 worlds: my life on the field as an athletic trainer and the research that was showing that some of our clinical practices were not always up to date. Since then, the research and information available to us has grown tremendously, and we have become leaders in determining how to best prevent and treat heat illnesses and prevent death from exertional heat stroke. As clinicians, we need to continue to not only be open minded and constant seekers of knowledge, but we must ensure that we are applying the latest evidence-based information into our clinical practice.

The information on how to prevent, recognize, and treat exertional heat illnesses is available via various avenues. This book provides the clinician with a hub of information to very common clinical questions as they pertain to various heat illnesses and hydration in exercising individuals. The responses to the 39 questions are based on the latest evidence and are presented in a way that is clinically applicable. The authors of the responses to these clinical questions are experts who have incorporated the most updated evidence-based information as well as their own personal experiences in the lab, clinic, on the field, and in medical tents. The book is divided into 5 sections: prevention, diagnosis, emergency management and treatment, special considerations regarding environment and return to play, and hydration. This book is intended as a resource for athletic trainers, students, and other health care professionals who are seeking the answers to the common questions we may have regarding exertional heat illnesses and hydration. The best way to use this resource is to skim through the Contents and select a question that you may have regarding heat-related illnesses, hydration, and other related topics. Each question has a stand-alone response that will quickly give you the facts and an explanation. I hope you find that this book is a great resource that can be used by clinicians in various settings.

Rebecca M. Lopez, PhD, ATC, CSCS
Assistant Professor
Department of Orthopaedics and Sports Medicine
Morsani College of Medicine
University of South Florida
Tampa, Florida

SECTION I

PREVENTION

WHAT ARE THE BASIC GUIDELINES FOR PREVENTING EXERTIONAL HEAT ILLNESSES, INCLUDING HEAT CRAMPS, HEAT SYNCOPE, HEAT EXHAUSTION, AND EXERTIONAL HEAT STROKE?

Riana R. Pryor, MS, ATC and
Douglas J. Casa, PhD, ATC, FACSM, FNATA

Many athletes suffer from exertional heat illnesses (EHI), especially when exercising in hot and humid environments. Although the causes of each type of illness are different, following a few preventative strategies can decrease the incidence of heat cramps, heat syncope, heat exhaustion, and exertional heat stroke. The goals of these preventative measures are to ensure that the body can thermoregulate at an optimal level and to gradually expose the body to extreme environments. Coaching and medical staff should work together to ensure that all safety precautions are in place prior to the start of a sports season (Figure 1-1).

Strategy 1: Heat Acclimatization

Adopting a heat-acclimatization protocol during the first 2 weeks of exercise is a strategy that can decrease the incidence of all types of heat illnesses. Heat acclimatization introduces the body to hot environments gradually, which helps induce beneficial changes to thermoregulatory and cardiovascular function.[1] Some of these

Lopez RM, ed. *Quick Questions in Heat-Related Illness and Hydration: Expert Advice in Sports Medicine* (pp 3-6).
© 2015 Taylor & Francis Group.

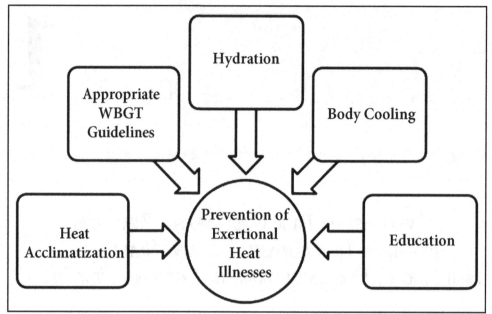

Figure 1-1. Following these prevention strategies can reduce the incidence of EHI.

changes include increased stroke volume, plasma volume, and sweat rate; faster onset of sweating; and decreased resting and exercising internal body temperature, heart rate, and sweat sodium concentration.[2] Combined, these physiological changes keep the body cooler in hot environments by improving heat tolerance and heat dissipation during exercise. Not only do these adaptations improve safety, but they also can improve athletic performance.

To see the greatest physiological changes, each exercise session should last at least 60 to 90 minutes in at least 25°C/77°F temperature. Over the course of the heat-acclimatization period, the duration and number of exercise sessions should increase, while additional clothing or equipment can be added gradually. Traditionally, practices lasting longer than 3 hours in the heat are not recommended, especially in the first few days of heat acclimatization because of increased risk of developing EHI. If multiple practices occur within 1 day, leave at least 3 hours between practices to allow time to rest, eat, hydrate, and allow the body to cool to resting temperatures.

Strategy 2: Wet Bulb Globe Temperature Considerations

The hottest part of the day (from 10 am until 3 pm) should be avoided when planning sporting events (including games, practices, and conditioning sessions).

By monitoring wet bulb globe temperature (WBGT), the school's medical staff can determine if games or practices should be postponed or modified because of extreme temperatures. The American College of Sports Medicine created WBGT guidelines[2] that outline when and how to modify exercise by introducing additional water breaks to decrease the work-to-rest ratio.[3] Recently, modified guidelines from evidence-based medicine have been established.[4] Specifically, if the WBGT rises above 28°C/82°F, all sports games and practices should be postponed. If this is not followed, medical staff should be on high alert that cases of EHI are likely. If these guidelines are followed, teams can keep athletes safe by decreasing the likelihood of developing an EHI.

Strategy 3: Hydration

Maintaining euhydration during exercise plays a key role in the prevention of EHI. As an individual exercises in hot environments, the body sweats to increase heat loss via evaporation. If the volume of sweat is not replaced with the same volume of fluid ingested, dehydration, which decreases stroke volume and strains the thermoregulatory system, occurs. For every 1% of body mass loss during exercise there is a 0.5°F increase in internal body temperature. If this happens, heat exhaustion and exertional heat stroke are more likely to result during exercise, and heat syncope may occur immediately upon cessation of exercise. To offset sweating during exercise, athletes should drink fluids to a minimum of 2% dehydration.

To increase accuracy with fluid consumption, athletes should undergo individualized sweat rate analysis by measuring body weight before and after exercise. Weight loss indicates fluid lost during the exercise session. Beginning exercise when hydrated is also an important way to prevent many types of EHI. To avoid hypohydration, athletes should monitor their urine color throughout the day. If urine is dark yellow instead of nearly clear, water should be consumed to achieve an optimal hydration level.

Extensive fluid and sodium losses through sweating, along with physical fatigue, have been proposed to predispose individuals to heat cramps. To prevent this disabling event, additional sodium in the diet or ingesting sodium during exercise could attenuate this condition. To fully understand the exact amount of sodium with which to supplement, the whole body wash-down technique can be used.[5] By understanding the amount of sodium that is excreted from the body during exercise, and analyzing the individual's diet for sodium, athletes can replace this exact amount with a premeditated hydration and sodium supplementation plan. For athletes without contraindications to increased sodium intake, this diet change can increase the amount of fluid retained in the body, allowing for greater blood volume and more effective body cooling.

Strategy 4: Body Cooling

Cooling before and during exercise, and between consecutive bouts of exercise, mitigates the rise in internal body temperature that occurs with muscular contraction. The most efficient modality of body cooling is cold-water immersion because of the large temperature gradient between cold water and the body. Some examples of less effective but portable cooling modalities include cold-water immersion of the hands and feet, ice towels, ice jackets, and ice slurry ingestion. Even a moderate decrease in internal body temperature (0.5°C) has been shown to improve performance while decreasing the risk of developing EHI.[6] Practical application, efficacy, and timing of cooling should be considered when determining an appropriate cooling modality.

Strategy 5: Education/Communication

Educating athletes and coaches on the signs and symptoms of EHI can be crucial in decreasing the severity of the condition if one arises. Athletes should ensure that they adjust to exercising in hot environments gradually and keep open communication with the coaching and medical staff to ensure that they stay safe and avoid EHI. When exercising with friends, athletes should let someone know if they begin to feel any symptoms of EHI or do not feel well. By adopting heat acclimatization and hydration plans and scheduling practice sessions during cooler parts of the day, teams can avoid the majority of complications due to EHI.

References

1. Pryor RR, Casa DJ, Adams WM, et al. Maximizing athletic performance in the heat. *Strength Cond J*. 2013;35(6):24-33.
2. Armstrong LE, Maresh CM. The indication and decay of heat acclimatization in trained athletes. *Sports Med*. 1991;12(5):302-312.
3. Armstrong LE, Casa DJ, Millard-Stafford M, Moran DS, Pyne SW, Robert WO. American College of Sports Medicine position stand: exertional heat illness during training and competition. *Med Sci Sports Exerc*. 2007;39(3):556-572.
4. Georgia High School Association, By-Law 2.67: Practice Policy for Heat and Humidity, 2013. www.ghsa.net/sites/default/files/documents/sports-medicine/HeatPolicy2013.pdf. Accessed May 25, 2013.
5. Shirreffs SM, Maughan RJ. Whole body sweat collection in humans: an improved method with preliminary data on electrolyte content. *J Appl Physiol*. 1996;82(1):336-341.
6. Tyler CJ, Sunderland C, Cheung SS. The effect of cooling prior to and during exercise on exercise performance and capacity in the heat: a meta-analysis. *Br J Sports Med*. 2013;0:1-8.

WHAT FACTORS LEAD TO EXERTIONAL HEAT STROKE?

Rebecca M. Lopez, PhD, ATC, CSCS

Exertional heat stroke (EHS) is a life-threatening condition that occurs when an exercising individual's heat gain has overpowered the body's ability to dissipate heat. EHS is characterized as having a dangerously elevated body temperature (> 104°F) along with central nervous system dysfunction.[1] The causes of EHS are multifactorial, with a combination of intrinsic and extrinsic factors playing a role (Table 2-1). Examples of intrinsic factors may include fitness level and an underlying illness, while extrinsic factors may include environmental conditions or protective equipment. When an exercising individual succumbs to EHS, it is often the result of several of these factors, and not one single predisposing factor. Although EHS may not always be preventable, being aware of the potential causes of EHS is imperative to decreasing the risk of EHS in exercising individuals.

Knowing that EHS is not caused by one factor alone is extremely important in decreasing the risk of this potentially catastrophic condition. Understanding these predisposing factors allows athletes, coaches, and health care professionals to minimize the risk. For instance, many individuals believe that hydration alone will

Lopez RM, ed. *Quick Questions in Heat-Related Illness and Hydration: Expert Advice in Sports Medicine* (pp 7-10).
© 2015 Taylor & Francis Group.

Table 2-1
Risk Factors for Exertional Heat Stroke

Intrinsic Factors	Extrinsic Factors
Poor physical fitness	Protective equipment
Sleep deprivation	Hot/humid environment
Improper acclimatization	Improper rehydration
Body composition	Exercise intensity
Underlying illness	Improper work-to-rest ratio
Medication	Physical effort unmatched to fitness level

prevent EHS. In an organized sport setting, such as a high school football team, a coach may allow athletes to hydrate during practice but may still place the football players at risk by not taking the other risk factors into consideration. Although there is a relationship between hydration and body temperature when exercising in the heat, staying hydrated does not entirely prevent EHS. A series[2] of 134 cases of heat strokes (6 of these fatal) outlined the many factors that contributed to each case of EHS. The athletes in the 6 fatal cases had an average of 11 predisposing factors (individual limitations, environmental factors, organization factors, and treatment factors) that led to their EHS and their deaths.[2] The athletes in the non-fatal cases of EHS had fewer than 5 factors recorded. Regardless of the outcome, it is evident that this condition is a result of a "perfect storm" of several risk factors. The risks can also vary by individual, whereby several individuals may be exposed to the same extrinsic risks but only one individual suffers an EHS. Therefore, it is essential for individuals and for those in charge of organizing athletic events to recognize both the intrinsic and extrinsic factors that can result in EHS, and steps should be taken to prevent them.

Although intrinsic factors may not always be modifiable, identifying the risk factors an athlete may have is the key to prevention. As the Rav-Acha et al[2] case series demonstrated, an exercising individual might have several intrinsic risk factors present. The most commonly cited intrinsic factors included having an underlying illness (fever or gastrointestinal distress), low physical fitness, sleep deprivation, being overweight, and dehydration. In fact, athletes in 5 out of the 6 fatal cases had low physical fitness, and 5 out of 6 experienced some level of sleep deprivation in the night(s) preceding the EHS.[2] Interestingly, in another case series of 10 EHS survivors, 7 out of the 10 patients had sleep loss as well.[3] This is important to note, as many exercising individuals may not be aware that sleep loss is a predisposing factor to heat stress.

An individual's level of heat acclimatization is also an important component of EHS prevention.[4] The process of being heat acclimatized, where the body physiologically adapts to exercising in the heat, plays a major role in how an individual's body will respond to the demands placed on it. A recent epidemiological study on the incidence of exertional heat illness among US high school athletes revealed that 60% of heat illnesses occurred in August; of these, over 90% occurred during preseason.[5] This further supports the need for adequate heat acclimatization policies and procedures for all levels of sport participation.

Being overweight or having a high body mass index is also commonly cited as a risk factor for EHS.[2,4,5] Body composition is often found in conjunction with poor physical fitness, which is another risk factor for EHS. When an individual with a poor fitness level is exercising alongside others who are more fit, this may lead to an increased exercise intensity in order to keep up and increases the risk of hyperthermia.[1] Certain medications (eg, antihistamines, calcium channel-blockers, amphetamines) have also been shown to increase the risk of EHS by impeding heat dissipation and/or increasing heat production.[3,4] The presence of an underlying illness, such as gastrointestinal distress or fever, has also been recorded in many cases of EHS.[2-4] If an individual presents with an illness associated with an elevated body temperature and/or dehydration prior to beginning exercise, this should preclude him or her from participating that day. Exercising while dehydrated has been shown to increase heart rate and body temperature when compared with a euhydrated individual exercising at the same intensity.[4]

Some of the extrinsic factors often cited as potential causes of EHS include environmental conditions, protective equipment, lack of rest breaks or improper work-to-rest ratios, and access to fluids, among others. Although not all extrinsic factors (such as the environment) are modifiable, other organizational factors can be.

Although EHS can occur in the absence of a hot and humid environment, extreme temperatures are often associated with a greater risk of heat illness. The 6 cases of fatal EHS in the Rav-Acha et al study[2] were associated with exercise or training in the presence of high solar radiation (5 out of 6), a wet bulb globe temperature $> 80.6°F$ (5 out of 6), and training during the hottest hours of the day (5 out of 6).[2] In particular, a high relative humidity can impede the body's ability to dissipate heat via evaporation of sweat and is often present in cases of EHS.[3] Improper work-to-rest ratios and physical effort unmatched to physical fitness seem to increase the risk of EHS as well.

Protective equipment, whether in the athletic or military setting, often increases heat load and impairs the body's ability to cool. This is further exacerbated with a decrease in the amount of exposed skin. Protective clothing in combination with poor body composition has also been found to further increase body temperature and fatigue during exercise in the heat.[4]

Most extrinsic factors associated with EHS are modifiable in some way. Organizational factors such as decreasing the amount of equipment worn, changing practice or exercise time to the cooler parts of the day, and employing appropriate work-to-rest cycles will help decrease the risk. The use of frequent rest breaks and adequate hydration, particularly when environmental conditions are harsh, are other means of altering the extrinsic risk factors for EHS.

Conclusion

Understanding the causes of EHS is the first step in prevention. It is imperative for clinicians to understand the various risk factors and determine ways to modify these risk factors in their clinical settings. Risk factors can vary by location and setting. Despite the common risk factors cited in the literature, the predisposing factors for EHS can also vary by individual. Education about the risk of exercising in the heat, pre-exercise screening, monitoring hydration status, and modifying organizational factors pertaining to work-rest cycles, equipment, and training time can help in the prevention of EHS.

References

1. Casa DJ, Guskiewicz KM, Anderson SA, et al. National Athletic Trainers' Association position statement: preventing sudden death in sports. *J Athl Train*. 2012;47(1):1-24.
2. Rav-Acha M, Hadad E, Epstein Y, Heled Y, Moran DS. Fatal exertional heat stroke: a case series. *Am J Med Sci*. 2004;328(2):84-87.
3. Armstrong LE, De Luca JP, Hubbard RW. Time course of recovery and heat acclimation ability of prior exertional heatstroke patients. *Med Sci Sports Exerc*. 1990;22(1):36-48.
4. Casa DJ, Armstrong LE, Kenny GP, O'Connor FG, Huggins RA. Exertional heat stroke: new concepts regarding cause and care. *Curr Sports Med Rep*. 2012;11(3):115-123.
5. Kerr ZY, Casa DJ, Marshall SW, Comstock RD. Epidemiology of exertional heat illness among U.S. high school athletes. *Am J Prev Med*. 2013;44(1):8-14.

WHAT ARE THE PHYSIOLOGICAL BENEFITS OF HEAT ACCLIMATIZATION?

Matthew S. Ganio, PhD

Heat acclimatization/acclimation is one of the most dramatic short-term changes the body can undergo. Repeated exposures to the heat over multiple days lead to cardiovascular and thermoregulatory adaptations that result in performance improvements and reductions in heat illnesses. Clinicians should assist athletes in taking advantage of this safe, legal, and natural process, which is relatively easy to employ. This section will explain the process of heat acclimatization, as well as how it affects the body, improves performance, and reduces the risk of heat illness.

Physiological Adaptations With Heat Acclimatization

Heat acclimatization invokes multiple adaptations of the cardiovascular and thermoregulatory systems. With heat acclimatization, blood volume (specifically plasma volume) increases anywhere between 3% and 27%.[1] This allows for

Lopez RM, ed. *Quick Questions in Heat-Related Illness and Hydration: Expert Advice in Sports Medicine* (pp 11-15).

Table 3-1	
Basic Physiological Adaptations With Heat Acclimatization	
Physiological Measure	**Exercise Response** **Post- Versus Pre-Heat Acclimatization**
Heart rate	Lower
Body temperature	Lower
Rating of perceived exertion	Lower
Sodium loss in sweat	Lower
Sodium loss in urine	Lower
Plasma volume	Increased at rest
Aerobic exercise performance	Improved
Sweat rate	Increased

a greater stroke volume, and thus a lower heart rate is needed to perform exercise (Table 3-1). This partly explains why the same exercise feels easier after heat acclimatization (ie, lower rating of perceived exertion). Heat acclimatization also results in a conservation of whole-body electrolytes. Specifically, there is less sodium chloride (ie, salt) lost via sweat and urine after heat acclimatization (see Table 3-1).

Thermoregulation, or the body's ability to control body temperature, is greatly enhanced with heat acclimatization. Specifically, heat acclimatization increases sweat rate (see Table 3-1) and allows for greater heat dissipation. This occurs partly because the stimulus to begin sweating occurs at a lower body temperature (ie, earlier sweat onset), and there is a greater increase in sweat rate for every increased degree of body temperature (ie, increased sweat sensitivity).[2] Consequently, with heat acclimatization the body can more efficiently and effectively dissipate heat, resulting in a lower exercising body temperature. Having a lower exercising body temperature can reduce the risk for heat illness and increase performance by delaying fatigue.

Implications of Heat Acclimatization on Performance and Heat Illness

The obvious question before undergoing a heat acclimatization protocol is this: Why should I heat acclimatize? As mentioned, the physiological adaptations that occur with heat acclimatization improve performance and reduce incidences of heat illness.[1] It has been known for decades that heat acclimatization allows for better performance in the heat. Performance improvements are greatest for exercise that relies primarily on aerobic metabolism (eg, endurance-type exercise). This is because aerobic exercise stresses the cardiovascular and thermoregulatory systems, which benefit most from heat acclimatization. This does not imply that other, more anaerobic types of exercise (eg, sprinting-type exercise) do not benefit from heat acclimatization, but the magnitude may not be as great. Improved performance can be defined as the ability to exercise for a longer time period when intensity is the same before and after heat acclimatization (ie, time-to-exhaustion test); it can also be defined as the ability to cover a certain distance faster or do more work in a given time period (ie, time-trial). Heat acclimatization most dramatically improves time-to-exhaustion in hot climates,[3] while time-trial performance can be improved in hot *and* cold climates.[4] Therefore, regardless of the type of performance, or if it's just practice, most athletes will benefit from being heat acclimatized. Given the relative ease, safety, and legality of heat acclimatization, it is surprising that more athletes do not take advantage of it for performance improvements.

Regardless of exercise type, heat acclimatization reduces the risk of most heat illnesses, such as heat cramps, heat syncope, heat exhaustion, and exertional heat stroke.[1] Just a few days of heat acclimatization dramatically lowers the incidence and risk of heat stroke. This is evidenced by the fact that most heat strokes occur in the first few days of a "heat wave" or during physical conditioning in the heat before acclimatization has taken place. This is why athletic governing bodies such as the National Collegiate Athletic Association have instituted heat acclimatization policies to improve athlete safety. Although the exact mechanism is unknown, it is believed that heat acclimatization lowers incidences of heat illnesses such as exertional heat stroke by allowing the body to more effectively cool itself through increased sweating.

The Process of Heat Acclimatization

The process of heat acclimatization takes approximately 7 to 14 days of repeated heat exposures. Repeated heat exposures on consecutive days are necessary to acclimatize; however, it can still occur if there are consecutive days without heat exposure (although the adaptations may take longer).[1,2] When defining heat exposure, the athlete should consider the length of time for each exposure and the intensity of activities performed during the exposure. There is not a standard, ideal length of time or exercise intensity for each exposure, but often 60 to 90 minutes of physical activity at 40% to 75% of maximal oxygen uptake (ie, maximal effort) in a hot environment is used in clinical settings. Taken together, the exercise time and intensity should be adjusted as the athlete becomes acclimatized. Early exposures should be shorter in length and at lower exercise intensities because the body will not be able to efficiently handle the heat. As the heat acclimatization process occurs, longer exposures at higher intensities will be possible.[1] For example, the first few exercise sessions in the heat may need to consist of light conditioning for only 30 minutes. As the week progresses, longer workouts at higher intensities will be better tolerated because acclimatization to the heat is occurring. It is important to not push individual athletes who are struggling with the heat; this only increases their chances of having a heat illness and does not benefit the heat acclimatization process.

The reason heat acclimatization occurs is because the body gets used to having an increased body temperature and learns to adapt so that body temperature will not increase as much in the future. It does this primarily by sweating more.[1] An important side note is that fluid ingestion should replace sweat losses during or soon after each heat exposure in order to maximize the heat acclimatization process.[2] This allows the body to adequately increase blood volume and confer the benefits of improved thermoregulation.

Full heat acclimatization to an environment requires repeated heat exposures in the same or similar environment in which the athlete will perform.[1,2] For example, if the athlete will be performing in a 95°F, 30% relative humidity environment, the athlete should acclimatize to that environment by repeated exposures to 95°F (or greater) and 30% relative humidity. Heat exposure in more temperate environments (eg, 80°F) will still incur some adaptations; however, full heat acclimatization to the harsher environment will not be incurred.

After acclimatization is achieved, the athlete will want to maintain the adaptations. Without continued heat exposure, the beneficial adaptations that have occurred will diminish over time, reverting to pre-acclimatization status. In order to maintain the adaptations, heat-acclimatized athletes are encouraged to have at least one heat exposure approximately every 6 days.[1]

The efficiency, time course, and magnitude of heat acclimatization that occurs among individuals may depend on physical parameters. There is some evidence that obese individuals may take longer to heat acclimatize and that the magnitude may not be as great.[5] After taking fitness differences into account, the process of heat acclimatization is not different among adults of different ages or gender,[1,2] but children (< 18 years old) may have less of an adaptation to the heat.

Conclusion

Heat acclimatization occurs most effectively when an athlete exercises for 60 to 90 minutes at a moderate intensity for 7 to 14 consecutive days in the heat. Heat acclimatization is a safe, legal process in which the cardiovascular and thermoregulatory systems beneficially adapt in a manner that improves performance and reduces heat illnesses.

References

1. Armstrong LE, Maresh CM. The induction and decay of heat acclimatisation in trained athletes. *Sports Med.* 2011;12(5):302-312.
2. Wenger CB. Human heat acclimatization. In: Pandolf KB, Sawka MN, Gonzalez RR, eds. *Human Performance Physiology and Environmental Medicine at Terrestrial Extremes*. Traverse City, MI: Benchmark Press; 1988:153-197.
3. Pandolf KB. Time course of heat acclimation and its decay. *Int J Sports Med.* 1998;19(suppl 2):S157-S160.
4. Lorenzo S, Halliwill JR, Sawka MN, Minson CT. Heat acclimation improves exercise performance. *J Appl Physiol.* 2010;109(4):1140-1147.
5. Dougherty KA, Chow M, Kenney WL. Responses of lean and obese boys to repeated summer exercise in the heat bouts. *Med Sci Sports Exer.* 2009;41(2):279-289.

References

WHAT ARE THE LATEST GUIDELINES FOR BECOMING HEAT ACCLIMATIZED AND BETTER PREPARED WHEN EXERCISING IN A WARM ENVIRONMENT?

Michelle A. Cleary, PhD, ATC

For optimal safety regardless of competition level, all coaches and athletes must follow current acclimatization guidelines that progressively increase training demands and exposure to environmental conditions.[1] Acclimatization is essential for any physically active individual preparing to exercise, train, or compete in a warm or humid environment to which he or she is unaccustomed. Athletes in equipment-intensive sports (for example, American football, lacrosse, and hockey) also need additional time to acclimatize to the uniform and to the intensity and duration of practice.[2] Most athletes, but American football players specifically, are at particularly greater risk during the early preseason, when the environment is often hotter and more humid and the uniform configuration and workload may be inappropriate for the level of fitness and acclimatization of individual players.[2] Several professional organizations, including the National Athletic Trainers' Association (NATA), the Korey Stringer Institute, and many states have developed best practice statements to guide heat acclimatization programs that emphasize safety for athletes conditioning in a warm environment.[1,3-5] According to the Korey

Lopez RM, ed. *Quick Questions in Heat-Related Illness and Hydration: Expert Advice in Sports Medicine* (pp 17-21).

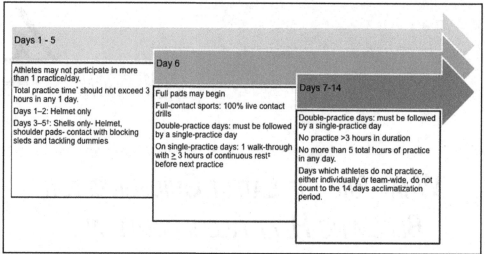

Figure 4-1. Recommendations for 14-day heat acclimatization period[4,5]
*Practice time includes warm-up, stretching, cool-down, walk-through, conditioning, and weight-room activities.
†If a practice is interrupted by inclement weather or heat restrictions, the practice should recommence once conditions are deemed safe.
‡Rest: At least 3 continuous hours resting in a cool environment.

Stringer Institute, there have been zero deaths in high school athletic programs in states that have passed heat acclimatization guidelines.[5] Smart implementation of a well-designed acclimatization program with appropriate oversight by an athletic trainer can dramatically enhance the safety of sport participation (Figure 4-1).[1]

A proper heat-acclimatization plan is essential to minimize the risk of exertional heat illness (EHI) during the preseason practice period or at any time an individual begins exercising in the heat.[4] Gradually increasing athletes' exposure to the duration and intensity of physical activity and to the environment minimizes the risk of EHI while improving athletic performance.[4] Any new exercise or training drill introduced into a strength-and-conditioning program should be added in a deliberate, gradual fashion over a 14-day period. This gradual progression is particularly important during the early stages of a conditioning program.[1,3] According to best practice guidelines proposed by the NATA and the Korey Stringer Institute, a gradual progression plan is especially important during the initial 3 to 5 days (see Figure 4-1) of summer practices.[1,3-5] The first 7 to 10 days (at minimum, the first 4 separate-day workouts) of any new conditioning cycle (including but not limited to return in January, after spring break, return in summer, and return after an injury) are referred to as transitional periods.[1,3] A written, progressive program of increasing volume, intensity, mode, and duration should be instituted for all transitional periods.[1,3] These conditioning programs should be approved by a credentialed strength and conditioning coach who should work cooperatively with medical staff (certified athletic trainer, team physician, or both) when developing transitional workout plans, particularly if the athlete is recovering from an injury or if any uncertainty exists regarding the pace of exercise progression.[3]

Although there are set guidelines that organized teams may follow, training and conditioning programs may need to be individualized because some athletes require a longer acclimatization process. An athlete at a different level of preparedness from his or her teammates (due to injury or time away from training) should use a training program tailored to his or her level.[3] A good starting place would emphasize recovery by incorporating conditioning programs during transitional periods that include a 1:4 work-to-rest ratio (with greater rest permissible) when conducting serial activity of an intense nature.[1,3] Integrating sport-specific drills, such as shuttle runs, agility drills, and short sprints at a high intensity, is an effective way to acclimatize aerobic and anaerobic sport teams to the heat. Four 30- to 45-minute sessions of this high intensity activity (approximately 75% VO_2max) over the course of 10 to 14 days in hot conditions are sufficient.[1,4,5]

Athletes participating in sports that require protective equipment such as football, lacrosse, and field hockey (ie, goalies) should avoid wearing protective equipment for the first 5 days of practice in a hot environment and then gradually add equipment to subsequent practices (see Figure 4-1). These athletes and nonacclimatized or aerobically unfit athletes should be introduced to single practice sessions for the first 5 days with succeeding practices alternating between single and double practice days (see Figure 4-1).[1] Coaches designing conditioning programs must identify individual athletes who may be at a different preparedness level and develop a training program tailored to their level of fitness or other medical needs.[3,4]

Conditioning periods should be phased in gradually and progressively to encourage proper exercise acclimatization and to minimize the risk of adverse effects on health (Table 4-1).[3] However, it is remarkable how few high school football programs respond to environmental heat stress with proven modifications such as adjustments to equipment use or practice activities during any part of their schedule, including preseason. Slightly more than 50% of high school football programs reported using a "helmets-only" and "no-pads" protocol in excessive heat, which suggests that many coaches and athletic directors may not appreciate the heat-injury risk associated with heat trapped by the football uniform.[2] Greater implementation of effective prevention measures to reduce the incidence of heat-related injury and death in high school American football is needed. Strategies should focus on modifying practices appropriately on a day-to-day basis to minimize heat strain and optimize hydration, identifying and educating at-risk individuals during the preparticipation period, and developing an emergency action plan for effectively managing heat injuries.[2]

Table 4-1
Heat Acclimatization Guidelines[1,5]

Introduce New Conditioning Activities Gradually

- New conditioning activities should be introduced gradually over a period of 14 days of exposure to warm or hot environments.
- During transition periods, conditioning activities should be phased in gradually and progressively to encourage proper exercise acclimatization and minimize the risk of adverse events.
- Include a progressive program of increasing volume, intensity, mode, and duration for all transitional periods.
- Utilize an appropriate work-to-rest ratio for the sport, especially during serial, intense activity.
- Allow sufficient recovery during training sessions.
- Training programs should be individualized. Some athletes require a longer acclimatization process.

Do Not Use Exercise and Conditioning Activities as Punishment

- No additional physical burden that would increase the risk of injury or sudden death should be placed on the athlete under any circumstance.[3]

Provide Appropriate Supervision and Medical Coverage

- Participation should be supervised by a qualified coach or credentialed individual who is knowledgeable about and uses acclimatization principles.
- All coaches or individuals conducting and/or supervising conditioning sessions must be prepared to provide first aid as soon as an athlete shows signs of distress.
- All coaches should be able to administer cardiopulmonary resuscitation, apply an automated external defibrillator, and activate the emergency action plan if needed.
- An athletic trainer or team physician should be present during each high-risk conditioning session.

Most importantly, transitional conditioning periods must be carefully conducted and supervised by medical personnel, such as an athletic trainer or an appropriately credentialed strength and conditioning coach with cardiopulmonary resuscitation and first-aid training. Further, under no circumstance should exercise and conditioning activities be used as punishment. Physical activity should not be used as retribution, for coercion, or as discipline for unsatisfactory athletic or academic performance or unacceptable behavior. No additional physical burden that would increase the risk of injury or sudden death should be placed on the athlete under any circumstance.[3] To be successful in preventing EHI or sudden death during training and conditioning in the heat, properly designed heat acclimatization policies must be developed, implemented, and followed. A well-designed heat acclimatization program requires 10 to 14 days of gradually progressive exercise with protective equipment. All individuals exercising in the heat must complete the heat acclimatization period regardless of time of arrival to preseason practice. Finally, having mandatory state guidelines for heat acclimatization provides a critical standard to protect athletes against EHI, and possibly saves lives.[5]

References

1. Casa DJ, Almquist J, Anderson SA, et al. The Inter-Association Task Force for preventing sudden death in secondary school athletics programs: best-practices recommendations. *J Athl Train*. 2013;48(4):546-553.
2. Luke AC, Bergeron MF, Roberts WO. Heat injury prevention practices in high school football. *Clin J Sports Med*. 2007;17(6):488-493.
3. Casa DJ, Anderson SA, Baker L, et al. The Inter-Association Task Force for preventing sudden death in collegiate conditioning sessions: best practices recommendations. *J Athl Train*. 2012;47(4):477-480.
4. Casa DJ, Csillan D, Armstrong LE, et al. Preseason heat-acclimatization guidelines for secondary school athletics. *J Athl Train*. 2009;44(3):332-333.
5. The Korey Stringer Institute. Heat acclimatization guidelines by state. http://ksi.uconn.edu/prevention-strategies/high-school-state-policies/heat-acclimatization-state-policies/. Accessed March 12, 2014.

IF AN ATHLETE LIVES IN A CONSTANTLY WARM ENVIRONMENT (EG, SOUTHERN PARTS OF THE UNITED STATES), IS HEAT ACCLIMATIZATION STILL AN ISSUE IN ATHLETIC PARTICIPATION?

Michele C. Benz, MS, ATC, CSCS and Rebecca M. Lopez, PhD, ATC, CSCS

Exertional heat stroke deaths continue to increase despite efforts in education and heat safety awareness.[1] With heat acclimatization as one of the most effective methods of preventing heat illness, athletes residing in both cool and warm climates should follow guidelines to ensure that their bodies have an adequate thermoregulatory response to exercise. When an athlete undergoes proper heat acclimatization, the body's response to exercise and heat is improved. Similarly, athletes not following a proper acclimatization program face measurable risks for heat illness.[2] Sweat rate, heart rate, and elevated core body temperature are all positively affected when athletes in any climate gradually take time to acclimate to hot conditions, whether dry or humid. The body then is able to maintain a lower core body temperature, drastically reducing the risk of exertional heat stroke and other heat illnesses. However, various factors affect both gaining and losing the physiological adaptations associated with heat acclimatization.

Lopez RM, ed. *Quick Questions in Heat-Related Illness and Hydration: Expert Advice in Sports Medicine* (pp 23-27).
© 2015 Taylor & Francis Group.

Although athletes in warmer climates may believe they acclimatize quickly, they need to gradually build exercise duration and intensity, especially during summer months when temperatures and relative humidity increase considerably. Research has shown that athletes are most at risk for heat illness during the first week of pre-season[1] because of increased environmental temperatures. However, temperatures throughout the year in many southern climates are on the rise, especially between September and February when exertional heat illnesses may not be a concern. In South Florida, for example, the average monthly temperature (AMT) and average maximum monthly temperature (AMMT) increased considerably during fall and winter.[3] From 1981 to 2010, the AMT between September and February was 74.2°F, and the AMMT was 81.3°F. In 2013, the AMT rose more than 2°F to 76.7°F, and the AMMT rose to 83.1°F.[3] When comparing the normal temperatures from 1981 to 2010 with those of recent years, there was a slight increase in temperature during summer months.[3]

In the southeastern United States, the heat index (indicative of air temperature and relative humidity) can often exceed 100°F in July and August, putting even the most seasoned athletes at risk for exertional heat stroke. A study observing the rate of exertional heat illnesses and the environmental conditions during a single football season in the Southeast reported that 123 out of 126 practices occurred during conditions considered to be of "high" or "extreme" risk.[4] In fact, 0 practices out of 126 during the entire season occurred during "no risk" conditions, with only 1 practice and 2 practices occurring during "low" and "moderate" risk conditions, respectively.[4]

This trend of rising temperatures indicates the need for athletes to acclimatize themselves prior to beginning their sport seasons, regardless of when their season takes place. To note, the heat index is taken in the shade, which may not be relevant to those exercising outdoors in the direct sunlight. The wet bulb globe temperature, which measures ambient temperature, relative humidity, and radiant heat from the sun, is the most accurate measurement of dangerous outdoor conditions for athletes and should be used to determine risk of heat illness. Using the wet bulb globe temperature allows clinicians to modify and supervise a safe heat acclimatization program.

Various physiological adaptations occur as athletes exercise in the heat, yet some factors may result in the loss of those adaptations. A typical heat acclimatization period is about 10 to 14 days prior to the start of the sport season. It is designed to ensure that exercising individuals go through a period of adjustment allowing the body to undergo the necessary metabolic changes to endure the stress of exercising in the heat. The heat acclimatization process prepares exercising individuals for these stressors and increases their ability to safely continue exercising.[1] Clinicians

Table 5-1 Decay of Heat Acclimatization	
Causes	**Effects**
Change in environmental conditions	Cardiovascular adaptations are lost
Inactivity due to injury or break in season	Elevated body temperature during exercise
Not exercising at a high enough intensity	Decreased sweat rate
Not exercising in hot and/or humid environment	Increased sweat sodium losses during exercise

should ensure that athletes who undergo periods of inactivity due to injury are able to reacclimatize prior to returning to full practices and competitions.

The decay or loss of heat acclimatization is extremely important in the athletic setting. Research has shown that the loss of some of these adaptations gained with heat acclimazation can occur in as little as a few days (Table 5-1), especially in athletes who partake in a very high volume and intensity of exercise.[5] Inactivity or activity in cooler climates, especially performing exercise that is not above 50% of the athlete's VO_2max, can reverse the acclimatization process. When this occurs, exercising heart rate will increase and stroke volume will decrease. Sweat rate and sweating onset will be drastically reduced, and perceived exertion will increase. These factors can result in an immediate increase in core and skin temperature responses and increase the risk of exertional heat illness.

The aerobic power of the athlete has been shown to determine the rate of decay of heat acclimatization.[5] Heat acclimatization decay was more significant in less fit athletes with lower aerobic power than their trained counterparts. Adaptations to heat stress took longer in untrained individuals, and the loss of acclimation was quicker. Factors that can lead to the decay of heat acclimatization can include inactivity due to being off-season or being injured, lower fitness levels, and changes in climate (ie, cold front followed by heat wave). Those exercising in the South during nonsummer months should continue to use caution because heat acclimatization policies and procedures are not usually in effect during this time.

Southern climates often face quickly changing temperatures, especially in the winter months. Cold fronts that drastically drop temperatures by as much as 25°F or 30°F can affect the body's adaptations to heat during the winter months, allowing for the decay of acclimatization of athletes. Therefore, if ambient conditions change drastically, as occurs when temperatures begin to cool and then rise suddenly, health care professionals should not assume that the athletes who had been

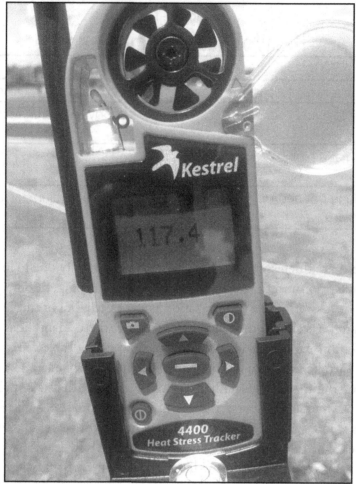

Figure 5-1. Example of elevated black globe temperature in the spring.

exercising in the cooler climate for some time are still heat acclimatized. Figure 5-1 illustrates an elevated black globe temperature measured in Florida in March, when the weather had been rather mild in the preceding days. In 2007, runners in the Chicago Marathon experienced an unexpected heat wave as temperatures reached extremes. Many of the runners appeared to be unprepared for those conditions, and the race was ultimately stopped. Although this was an unusual circumstance, athletic trainers need to be cognizant of similar, unexpected changes in weather and how this may place their athletes at greater risk.

Another factor to consider in terms of heat acclimatization is that nowadays many young athletes spend less time outdoors in the off-season than their predecessors. This lack of heat exposure and exercise in warmer temperatures results in a greater need for heat acclimatization. If a high school cross country runner stayed indoors during the summer months and began running with the team in August, he or she would not be able to dissipate heat efficiently unless undergoing a proper 10- to 14-day acclimatization period. Therefore, the fact that an athlete may reside in a warm climate does not guarantee adequate heat acclimatization. Proper steps should be taken to ensure that an athlete goes through the necessary steps to elicit the physiological adaptations needed to safely exercise in the heat. The maintenance of these physiological adaptations is also paramount, particularly in climates with fluctuating environmental conditions.

It is imperative that all athletes undergo a heat acclimatization period prior to starting *any* sport season. This vital adjustment period will allow the body to gradually respond to intense exercise in hot and humid conditions. This will result in better heat dissipation, increased cardiac output, decreased heat storage from contracting muscles, and an increased sweat rate.[1] Finally, it is essential for athletic trainers and other health care professionals to take into account changes in weather conditions or prolonged periods of inactivity due to injury. It may be necessary to instill a period of heat acclimatization at times when it is not mandated in order to prevent the decay of heat acclimatization and decrease the risk of heat illness.

References

1. Casa DJ, et al. National Athletic Trainers' Association position statement: exertional heat illnesses. *J Athl Train.* 2015;50.
2. Casa DJ, Csillan D, Armstrong LE, et al. National Athletic Trainers' Association consensus statement: pre-season practice guidelines for high school athletics. *J Athl Train.* 2009;44(3):332-333.
3. National Oceanic and Atmospheric Administration. www.noaa.gov. Accessed March 6, 2014.
4. Cooper ER, Ferrara MS, Broglio SP. Exertional heat illnesses and environmental conditions during a single football season in the Southeast. *J Athl Train.* 2006;41(3):332-336.
5. Armstrong LE, Maresh CM. The induction and decay of heat acclimatization in trained athletes. *Sports Med.* 1991;12(5):302-312.

WHAT CAUSES HEAT CRAMPS AND HOW CAN THEY BE PREVENTED?

Rebecca L. Stearns, PhD, ATC and Deanna M. Dempsey, MS

Heat cramps are often characterized by painful, involuntary muscle spasms or muscle cramps during or after fatiguing exercise. These usually occur in the legs, and are different from muscle cramps in that they are associated with exercise in the heat when athletes have been sweating profusely. There are 2 main theories as to why cramping occurs in athletes. The classical view is described well by Bergeron[1] and Eichner.[2] This theory describes the mechanism being due to electrolyte loss, specifically sodium, via sweating. This view describes the condition of heat cramping. The second view explains that cramping can be due to muscular fatigue and overload.[3] This is commonly referred to as exercise-associated muscle cramping (EAMC). While there is evidence to support both theories, and the potential exists for contributing factors to be associated with EAMC and heat cramps, this chapter will focus on the classical view of heat cramps.

In the classical view of heat cramps, the cause is usually due to large electrolyte loss. Additionally, athletes who are "salty sweaters" and those who exercise for an extended duration or at a greater intensity than normal are at particular risk for

Lopez RM, ed. *Quick Questions in Heat-Related Illness and Hydration: Expert Advice in Sports Medicine* (pp 29-32).
© 2015 Taylor & Francis Group.

large salt losses, especially if no attempt is made to replace the salt during exercise.[1] Sweat losses may be enhanced by extended exercise, heat acclimatization, and exercise in hot environments. Increases in the amount of fluid lost can cause decreases in the athlete's overall blood volume and blood sodium levels, especially with excessive fluid (specifically water).

Athletes who are at risk include the following:

- Athletes who are not acclimatized to the heat (and therefore may not retain sweat sodium losses as effectively)

- Athletes who wear additional protective equipment or clothing

- Athletes who have multiple practice sessions in a day, consecutive days of strenuous exercise, or both (thus increasing total sweat loss potential)

- Athletes who dilute their sodium via copious amounts of water consumption[1]

The reason excessive salt loss can be problematic is explained by the diverse functions of sodium throughout the body. Sodium plays a large role in the regulation of fluids between cells and compartments via the sodium-potassium pump. Sodium also contributes to retention of fluids in the kidneys at the distal convoluted tubule of the nephron.[1] A decrease in interstitial space, from any of the fluid loss mechanisms listed earlier, places a greater compression upon the nerves themselves, causing hyperexcitability and initiation of action potentials for contraction.[1] This theory is supportive of a whole body decrease in sodium, and therefore muscle cramping may be diffuse. However, this theory does not address why athletes with hyponatremia do not classically present with muscle cramping.

The second theory on why heat cramps occur is that muscle fatigue and overload cause the muscle to cramp. Schwellnus and colleagues first proposed this theory in 1997[3] as a result of observations in EAMC cases that did not involve the classical signs/history consistent with electrolyte losses or that did not occur in hot environments. Therefore, the authors proposed that another factor was causing these cramps. Schwellnus et al hypothesized that "EAMC is caused by sustained abnormal spinal reflex activity which appears to be secondary to muscle fatigue. Local muscle fatigue is therefore responsible for increased muscle spindle afferent and decreased Golgi tendon organ afferent activity."[3] In such cases, cramping would be more localized to the specific fatigued muscle.

Though no clear mechanism has been defined, there is evidence to support both theories. In addition, human physiology has been consistently shown to be redundant in its pathways and processes. Therefore, many pathways and processes may lead to a similar result or place regulatory control over an outcome. In an examination of all of the body's regulation mechanisms, it is very rare that one mechanism or factor is solely responsible for an outcome.

Recent literature has examined both of these potential mechanisms. Jung et al[4] examined the effect of hydration and electrolyte supplementation on the ability to prevent muscle cramping. Subjects performed a calf-fatiguing protocol to induce muscle cramps. There were 2 trials in which subjects either consumed a carbohydrate beverage with sodium added or they were not allowed to consume any fluids. The authors concluded that consuming the carbohydrate beverage in a hot environment more than doubled the time to cramping compared with the trial with no fluid consumption. However, about 70% of the subjects still had cramping, even when they consumed the carbohydrate beverage. This suggests that a carbohydrate beverage may delay but not completely prevent cramping from occurring.

Another study by Schwellnus et al[5] examined 210 ironman triathletes and found that the development of muscle cramping was associated with faster race times and not dehydration or serum electrolyte balance (suggesting that intensity was a greater factor than electrolyte balance). A challenge to any study examining muscle cramping, however, is the measurement of whole body sodium losses. Plasma sodium may be used to reflect fluid shifts in compartments (usually the movement of sodium into or out of cell walls); however, over long exercise durations it is not reflective of whole body sodium losses; therefore, studies that use this method to report sodium losses may not be entirely accurate.

In all, multiple mechanisms for muscle cramping exist, and different types of cramping can potentially occur. While some causes of cramping have been identified, the potential of other still unknown mechanisms is possible. See Table 6-1 for a summary of heat cramping theories and predisposing factors.

Based on current literature, the best recommendations to prevent muscle cramping for athletes follow:

- Acclimatize athletes to warm/hot environments (which will assist in retaining sweat sodium losses).

- Educate athletes to replace fluids appropriately and work to help athletes understand their hydration needs by measuring and explaining why it is important to minimize body mass losses or gains to less than 2%; also explain how athletes can measure their sweat rate in order to understand their individual fluid needs during exercise.

- In conjunction with understanding fluid needs, athletes who may experience recurrent issues with cramping may benefit from a full diet and sweat electrolyte analysis to determine if electrolytes are being appropriately replaced.

- Supplement the workout with electrolyte drinks if you anticipate the session to last more than 1 hour, if there are multiple bouts of exercise in the same day, if the athletes have not yet acclimatized to a warm environment, or if the athletes have a history of cramping or know they are considered a "salty sweater."

Table 6-1
Summary of 2 Theories Regarding Cause and Treatment for Heat Cramps

Cause	Theory 1[1,2] Sodium Loss	Theory 2[3,5] Muscular Fatigue
Mechanisms and Predisposing Factors	• Excessive sweating • Excessive water intake • Heat exposure • "Salty sweater" • Long exercise duration • Lack of heat acclimatization • Protective equipment or clothing	• Muscle fatiguing exercise (including short and long exercise bouts; fatigue is relative to exercise intensity over a period of time)
Treatment	• Consume sodium • Determine causative factors and implement preventative measures	• Passive stretching

• Train appropriately for the anticipated race/competition to avoid unique stressors on that day.

Given the current information on muscle cramps, it is impossible to determine a method to completely avoid muscle cramping but, as with any medical condition, if a muscle cramp does occur, it is important to take into account all the potential factors leading up to that event and modify those factors in order to reduce the incidence of future muscle cramps.

References

1. Bergeron MF. Muscle cramps during exercise: is it fatigue or electrolyte deficit? *Curr Sports Med Rep.* 2008;7(4):S50-S55.
2. Eichner ER. The role of sodium in "heat cramping." *Sports Med.* 2007;37:368-370.
3. Schwellnus MP, Derman EW, Noakes TD. Aetiology of skeletal muscle "cramps" during exercise: a novel hypothesis. *J Sport Sci.* 1997;15:277-285.
4. Jung AP, Bishop PA, Al-Nawwas A, et al. Influence of hydration and electrolyte supplementation on incidence and time to onset of exercise-associated muscle cramps. *J Athl Train.* 2005;40(2):71-75.
5. Schwellnus MP, Drew N, Collins M. Increased running speed and previous cramps rather than dehydration or serum sodium changes predict exercise-associated muscle cramping: a prospective cohort study in 210 ironman triathletes. *Br J Sports Med.* 2011;45(8):650-656.

What Is the Best Way to Prevent an Athlete From Overheating When Exercising in a Hot Environment?

Rebecca L. Stearns, PhD, ATC

Athletes exercising in hot environments gain heat through active muscle contractions and the surrounding environment, especially when the environment is above skin temperature. Because performance is improved and the risk of heat illness is decreased when body temperature remains lower, it is important to consider ways to mitigate these rises in body temperature. While hydration and heat acclimatization are 2 main strategies for optimizing the body's ability to cope with heat, this section will focus on acute cooling methods that can be used prior to or in between bouts of exercise in conjunction with a hydration or acclimatization strategy. It should be noted that this chapter deals with cooling for prevention and/or improving performance, rather than cooling for the sake of treating an exertional heat illness.

The 2 primary considerations for precooling or cooling between bouts of exercise are the amount of time available and the uniform or equipment load that the athlete needs to use. Football players will be restricted by the protective equipment they wear, as opposed to a runner or soccer player who may have very minimal

Lopez RM, ed. *Quick Questions in Heat-Related Illness and Hydration: Expert Advice in Sports Medicine* (pp 33-37).

barriers to cooling devices. The list of options for cooling is displayed in Table 7-1, in conjunction with potential disadvantages, reported cooling rates, and cooling potential if the method is applied for 5 minutes.

For athletes who are not limited by equipment, incorporation of water immersion or water dousing will result in the greatest cooling rates, and will therefore result in the greatest ability to keep an athlete cool before or in between bouts of exercise. For example, water immersion would be appropriate during the 30 minutes before exercise begins or for a soccer player during a 15-minute half time. In this second scenario, if the soccer player is able to cool for just 5 minutes in a very cold ice water immersion tub, he or she could potentially lower his or her body temperature by 3°F. This requires a tub or a pool that is large enough to immerse the athlete up to the shoulders in water, and would consequently also mean the athlete would need time to change clothes before heading back out to the game or practice. Many times a 150-gallon stock tank, which can fit 2 athletes at one time, will be used as an immersion tub. In any immersion scenario, there will be a large requirement for water and a lot of ice, but the cooling rates and overall benefit will be greater than other methods.

When athletes do not have access to a tub or large water source but are looking for a moderate degree of cooling, wet ice towels are a great alternative. These are also viable for athletes who use intensive equipment. Ice towels should be kept in coolers with a large amount of ice and water to cover the towels. When using the towels, they should be rotated roughly every 2 minutes to maintain an optimal gradient between the skin and cold towel. For optimum efficacy, towels should be placed over as much of the body as possible, such as the head, neck, chest, arms, legs, and feet. With aggressive ice-towel cooling, athletes could lower their body temperatures by as much as 1°F in 5 minutes. Ice towels also allow portability for the athlete while cooling and, depending on whether the entire body is covered in towels or not, they may not require a change of clothes. Lastly, ice vests have also been widely studied for athletes, and have suggested a small cooling effect, though the literature is debated.[1]

Other cooling modalities listed in Table 7-1 do not provide cooling rates that compare to these first 2 methods. There is the potential and additional literature to support the combination of 2 types of cooling, but even under such circumstances cold-water immersion (or extensive dousing) and wet ice towels are considered the leaders when it comes to cooling rates. In some scenarios athletes may not need a large drop in body temperature. For example, if the goal is to precool or prevent an athlete from overheating during exercise, these other cooling options may provide viable alternatives.

In addition to external cooling methods, a relatively new method, ice slurry ingestion, which cools internally, has demonstrated some promising results. In

Table 7-1

Various Cooling Modalities, Cooling Rates, and Potential Disadvantages

Cooling Method	Disadvantages	Advantages	Body Temperature Drop After 5 Minutes of Cooling
Cold-water immersion	Not practical for large groups, soaks clothing	Fastest cooling rates, cost effective	0.75°C to 1.75°C (1.35°F to 3.20°F)[2]
Cold-water dousing with ice massage	Not practical for large groups, soaks clothing	Fast cooling rates, immersion tubs not necessary, cost effective	0.70°C (1.26°F)[2]
Ice-wet towels*	Must constantly keep towels cold, soaks clothing	Moderate cooling rates, immersion tub not necessary, cost effective	0.55°C (1.00°F)[2]
Cold IV fluids*	Invasive, medical expertise required, may not be practical	Moderate cooling rates, improves hydration status if warranted	0.38°C (0.86°F)[2]
Cold-water splashing	Not practical for large groups, soaks clothing	Minimal water requirements, cost effective	0.22°C (0.40°F)[2]
Fanning only	Slower cooling rates	Large fans can be used for groups of athletes, easy application, does not soak clothes	0.01°C (0.02°F) 0.37°C (0.68°F)[2]
Cooling blankets	Slower cooling rates, high cost per athlete	Does not soak clothes	0.038°C (0.07°F)[2]
Ice packs on major arteries	Slow cooling rates	Easy application, cost effective	0.14°C (0.25°F)[2]

(continued)

Table 7-1 (continued)
Various Cooling Modalities, Cooling Rates, and Potential Disadvantages

Cooling Method	Disadvantages	Advantages	Body Temperature Drop After 5 Minutes of Cooling
Ice vest	Slow cooling rates, may be expensive for larger groups	Can be worn during a warm-up to limit body temperature rise	0.03°C (0.05°F)[1]
Ice slurry ingestion*	Requires special equipment, time to ingest fluid	Large appeal to athletes, does not require athlete to change clothes	N/A (0.66°C/7.5 g·kg⁻¹ bolus)[3]

*Practical for equipment intensive sports

this method, athletes ingest a given amount of ice slurry (which usually has the composition of a sports drink) about 30 minutes prior to exercise. This has resulted in a cooling effect of 1.2°F in 30 minutes.[3,4] This provides a very easy method of cooling for the athlete. However, if a flavored beverage is desired (to make it more similar to that of a frozen sports drink), purchasing these specialized drinks or the equipment to make them could be expensive. While no research has been done on homemade versions of these beverages, it is likely that they could have similar results.

Overall, the benefits of precooling can be great. In a recent systematic review with meta-analysis by Wegmann et al,[5] it was found that moderate effects associated with precooling strategies and performance outcomes were similar within intermittent sprint activity and endurance exercise. However, the greatest and largest effect reported for performance benefits from precooling was within a study utilizing endurance exercise performance outcomes. When types of precooling strategies were examined, water application had the greatest effect, followed by cold drinks. In total it was found that precooling of any kind, in any performance type, had an average increase in performance of 4.9%. In hot environments, this performance benefit was only exaggerated further.

Conclusion

Many different cooling strategies exist for athletes, and many new devices are created every day. A proper hydration regimen and adequate heat acclimatization are essential in preventing athletes from overheating while exercising in hot environments. However, for the purposes of precooling or cooling between bouts of exercise, the modalities that incorporate some use of cold water have consistently demonstrated higher cooling rates and therefore the greatest potential to keep hot athletes cooler, to minimize risk for heat illness, and to maximize performance in the heat.

References

1. Lopez RM, Zuri R, Jones L, Cleary MA. Effects of a cooling vest on core and skin temperature following a heat stress trial in healthy males. *J Athl Train.* 2008;43:55-61.
2. McDermott BP, Casa DJ, Ganio MS, et al. Acute whole-body cooling for exercise-induced hyperthermia: a systematic review. *J Athl Train.* 2009;44(1):84-93.
3. Siegel R, Mate J, Brearley MB, Watson G, Nosaka K, Laursen PB. Ice slurry ingestion increases core temperature capacity and running time in the heat. *Med Sci Sport Exerc.* 2010;42(4):717-725.
4. Siegel R, Mate J, Watson G, Nosaka K, Laursen PB. Pre-cooling with ice slurry ingestion leads to similar run times to exhaustion in the heat as cold water immersion. *J Sport Sci.* 2012;30(2):155-165.
5. Wegmann M, Faude O, Poppendieck W, Hecksteden A, Frohlich M, Meyer T. Pre-cooling and sports performance: a meta-analytical review. *Sport Med.* 2012;42(7):545-564.

WHAT IMPACT DOES PROTECTIVE EQUIPMENT (IE, HELMETS, PADDING) HAVE ON HEAT TOLERANCE?

Michelle A. Cleary, PhD, ATC

Sports requiring protective equipment (eg, American football, lacrosse, baseball catchers, hockey) with athletes who train and compete in warm weather have potential for serious and often life-threatening exertional heat stroke (EHS). This chapter describes how heat tolerance is affected by protective equipment that impedes cooling via evaporation, increases metabolic heat production via increased workload, and requires physiological adaptations to improve heat tolerance. Heat tolerance is the capacity for physical activity in the heat and depends on a delicate balance between heat absorbed from the environment, metabolic heat generated by muscles, and heat that is lost into the environment by evaporation of sweat from the skin. Exercise time decreases and heat absorbed by the body increases when there is a high ambient air temperature and moderate-to-high relative humidity, when exercise is intense, and when equipment is worn (Figure 8-1).[1] In order to best tolerate heat while wearing protective equipment, an athlete must either exercise less intensely or give the body time to adjust to exercise in hot environments by allowing time to acclimatize.

Lopez RM, ed. *Quick Questions in Heat-Related Illness and Hydration: Expert Advice in Sports Medicine* (pp 39-43).
© 2015 Taylor & Francis Group.

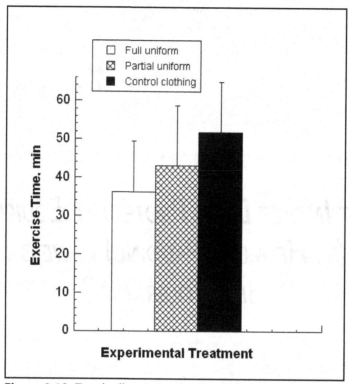

Figure 8-1A. Treadmill exercise time (mean ± SD) while wearing 3 clothing types (N = 10). The full uniform condition was less than the control clothing condition ($P = .002$, $d = 1.17$). The partial uniform condition was less than the control clothing condition ($P = .01$, $d = 0.59$) and greater than the full uniform condition ($P = .04$, $d = 0.48$). (Reprinted with permission from Armstrong LE, Johnson EC, Casa DJ, et al. The American football uniform: uncompensable heat stress and hyperthermic exhaustion. *J Athl Train*. 2010;45[2]:117-127.)

Heat tolerance is reduced when non–heat-acclimatized individuals fail to pay attention to warm-weather warnings, become dehydrated, or do not adapt their equipment to allow heat loss from the body.[2] The biophysical heat exchange between an exercising human and the environment is predictably modified by clothing systems according to the proportion of the body surface area covered, characteristics of the fabrics and protective materials, and the air trapped within and between material layers.[3] Depending on the characteristics of the fabric and materials, protective equipment reduces heat loss, as the materials are usually heavy, padded, and made of plastic that does not allow sweat to evaporate and cool the skin. Heat dissipation is reduced because the skin is covered and sweat cannot evaporate.[1] Clothing insulation increases as the percentage of the body surface area covered with garments increases and as the thickness of the garment layers increases.[3] The

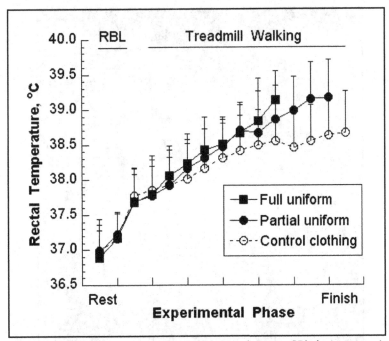

Figure 8-1B. Rectal temperature responses (mean ± SD) during repetitive box lifting, recovery, and treadmill exercise while wearing 3 different clothing types. Data points depict only those segments with 5 or more participants. (Reprinted with permission from Armstrong LE, Johnson EC, Casa DJ, et al. The American football uniform: uncompensable heat stress and hyperthermic exhaustion. *J Athl Train.* 2010;45[2]:117-127.)

evaporative resistance of equipment ensembles depends on the moisture permeability characteristics and wicking properties of the component materials and the amount of skin surface covered by those materials. Hard solid materials (used in helmets and shoulder pads) and foam padding, with or without a vinyl covering, particularly impede the evaporation of sweat (Figure 8-2).[3] In addition, the padding in the hips and legs is tight fitting, minimizing air circulation between the skin and the clothing. Football uniforms with the most body surface coverage have the lowest permeability, whereas practice uniforms (and t-shirt/shorts ensembles) provide the highest permeability, primarily because these lighter ensembles have the highest exposed body surface area for unimpeded evaporation of sweat.[3]

Uniforms for a variety of sports consist of protective equipment that contribute significantly to the heat load on a player,[3] reducing heat tolerance. Other than football, athletes playing lacrosse and goal keepers in soccer and field hockey, for example, often wear additional protective equipment, too. Adding this heavy or extensive protective equipment increases heat load on the body because of the extra weight and because it acts as a barrier to evaporation and cooling.[3] The thermal

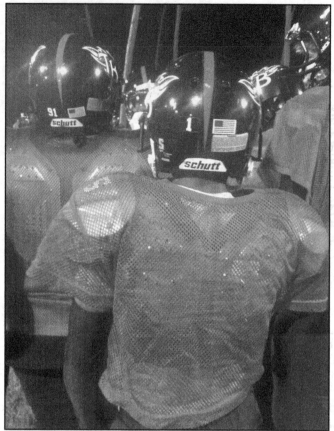

Figure 8-2. Example of an American football uniform.

and evaporative resistance of vapor-impermeable or plastic equipment adds to the heat storage and creates an added physiological challenge.[3] A variety of uniform ensembles have been researched[1-3] to determine that the primary contribution of wearing a helmet plus shoulder pads increases the rate of heat storage and reduces exercise-heat tolerance.[1] Compared with shorts only and practice uniforms, the pants in the full gear ensembles allow even less skin surface for evaporation and drive the core temperature up faster in less extreme environments.[2] Research[1] has demonstrated significant increases in heart rate, skin temperature, and rectal temperatures (see Figure 8-2) with different configurations of football equipment (full equipment, "shells," shoulder pads and helmet, and helmet only). Further, the weight of a football uniform increases metabolic rate, which increases heat production, and the inherent insulation of the rigid plastic and foam reduces heat dissipation to the surrounding air, decreasing heat loss.[2,3] To avoid EHS and to improve heat tolerance, athletes should wear no helmet or shoulder pads during the initial days of summer training.[1]

Participation guidelines recognize that athletes wearing protective equipment must take added precautions to avoid EHS when exercising in hot environments.[4] Although athletic equipment is needed for protection, preseason practices increase in intensity with the addition of protective equipment. To minimize the risk of adverse effects on health and maximize performance in the heat, protective equipment should be phased in gradually and progressively to encourage proper exercise acclimatization and improve heat tolerance.[4] Transition periods where acclimatization occurs are the first 7 to 10 days of any new conditioning cycle and should include gradual increases in the amount of equipment worn. Transitioning into any exercise in the heat includes, but is not limited to, returning to a sport in January, after spring break, return in summer, and return after time off due to an injury. During these potentially dangerous periods, cooperation with the medical staff (certified athletic trainer, team physician, or both) is particularly important if the athlete is recovering from an injury or if any uncertainty exists regarding the pace of exercise progression.[4] Following preseason training guidelines and gradually phasing in protective equipment after the initial acclimatization period are best practices to improve heat tolerance.[1,4]

Since full equipment ensembles, including helmet and shoulder pads, result in greater physiologic strain and shorter time to exhaustion, athletes should follow research findings[1] and organizational guidelines[4] that limit the use of a helmet and shoulder pads during the initial days of summer workouts to reduce the risk of EHS.[1,5] Considering every athlete's need for ample time to acclimatize in the heat, there is no justification for the traditional wearing of protective equipment during the initial 3 to 5 days of summer workouts, when the highest incidence of EHS occurs.[1] Therefore, to prevent EHS or other heat illnesses in any sport requiring protective equipment, it is important to reduce exercise intensity, include more frequent rest breaks, and increase hydration when environmental conditions are dangerous, particularly when protective equipment is worn.

References

1. Armstrong LE, Johnson EC, Casa DJ, et al. The American football uniform: uncompensable heat stress and hyperthermic exhaustion. *J Athl Train*. 2010;45(2):117-127.
2. Kulka TJ, Kenney WL. Heat balance limits in football uniforms how different uniform ensembles alter the equation. *Phys Sportsmed*. 2002;30(7):29-39.
3. McCullough EA, Kenney WL. Thermal insulation and evaporative resistance of football uniforms. *Med Sci Sports Exerc*. 2003;35(5):832-837.
4. Casa DJ, Anderson SA, Baker L, et al. The Inter-Association Task Force for preventing sudden death in collegiate conditioning sessions: best practices recommendations. *J Athl Train*. 2012;47(4):477-480.
5. Yeargin SW, Casa DJ, Armstrong LE, et al. Heat acclimatization and hydration status of American football players during initial summer workouts. *J Strength Cond Res*. 2006;20(3):463-470.

SHOULD ATHLETES STILL TAKE REST BREAKS EVEN IF THEY HAVE ACCESS TO FLUIDS THROUGHOUT ACTIVITY?

J. Luke Pryor, MS, ATC, CSCS and Riana R. Pryor, MS, ATC

On the surface, rest periods during physical activity appear to be used for the sole purpose of rehydrating to avoid dehydration. Following this logic, if athletes have access to fluids throughout activity, then rest or "hydration" breaks are not required. However, even when fluids are readily available during physical activity, voluntary fluid consumption by some athletes consists of only half of their body mass loss. This difference in body mass is primarily attributed to fluid loss resulting in voluntary dehydration.[1] For every percentage decrease in body mass due to dehydration, the rate of body temperature rise during exercise can increase up to ~0.25°C above rates of euhydrated individuals.[1] Moreover, if exercise intensity is high or environmental conditions are extreme, body temperature will rise despite adequate fluid intake during activity. Thus, the risks of dehydration and/or hyperthermia increase when rest periods are not taken during physical activity. It is well established that dehydration and/or hyperthermia increase the risk for exertional heat illness and reduce sport performance.[2-4] It is clear that rest breaks during physical activity are key components in the prevention of dehydration, performance decrements, and heat-related injury.[2]

Lopez RM, ed. *Quick Questions in Heat-Related Illness and Hydration: Expert Advice in Sports Medicine* (pp 45-48).
© 2015 Taylor & Francis Group.

There are several important physiological rationales for planning rest breaks into bouts of exercise, which contribute to improved physical performance and reduced heat-related injury risk. The physiological mechanisms underpinning the rise or fall in body temperature explain, in part, the need for rest breaks even if fluid is available during activity. Mathematically, we can present the relationship between whole-body heat gain and loss using the following heat balance equation:

$$S = M - (\pm W) \pm E \pm R \pm C \pm K$$

where S = heat storage, M = metabolic heat production, W = work, E = evaporation, R = radiation, C = convection, and K = conduction. Evaporation, radiation, convection, and conduction are heat transfer pathways that usually reduce thermal load, while metabolic heat production contributes only to heat gain. However, radiation, convection, and conduction can be positive, meaning that heat is stored by the body rather than dissipated when ambient air temperature is greater than body temperature. Simply put, if more heat is produced than lost, body temperature rises. Conversely, if less heat is produced than dissipated, body temperature decreases.

During intense physical activity, whole-body metabolism (ie, M) can be up to 20 times greater than resting levels.[3] The human metabolic system is only 20% efficient at utilizing chemical energy. The remaining 80% is given off as metabolic heat. This metabolic heat must be dissipated through the heat-loss mechanisms mentioned earlier or body temperature could rise to catastrophic levels very early in the exercise bout (104°F within 15 minutes).[3] A combination of factors dictate the rise in body temperature, including exercise-induced metabolic heat production, environmental conditions, and wearing clothes and equipment that impair evaporative heat loss transfer via sweating (eg, American football or military gear). Rest periods during exercise bouts help to mitigate the rise in body temperature by temporarily reducing metabolic heat production.

To maximize the effectiveness of reducing body temperature, efforts should be made to augment heat-loss mechanisms during rest periods. For example, resting in the shade (where ambient temperatures are usually lower) increases the temperature gradient between the body and the environment, thereby increasing radiative heat loss. Resting in the shade also reduces heat gain from solar radiation. Excess gear should be removed, if possible, and mechanical or manual fanning initiated to improve convective and evaporative heat loss.

Intense exercise alone, or in combination with hot environmental conditions, increases anaerobic metabolism. Anaerobic metabolism produces higher concentrations of metabolic by-products such as lactate and depletes muscle glycogen stores sooner compared with less intense exercise and/or cooler temperatures. The combined metabolic changes under these conditions, despite fluid access, negatively affect physical performance. For example, we recently demonstrated in euhydrated college-aged males that the number of boxes lifted over repeated, 10-minute bouts was significantly reduced in hot versus cool conditions (boxes lifted: 95 and 109, respectively).[4] Further, blood lactate concentrations were significantly higher in the hot versus cool conditions. From this perspective, rest periods are needed to reduce metabolic heat and lactate production. During rest breaks, lactate is cleared from the exercising muscle and circulation, and energy reserves are restored (intramuscular ATP, phosphocreatine, and glycogen). Appropriate work-rest cycles have been developed and are recommended by several organizational bodies to mitigate exertional heat injury and enhance physical performance when environmental conditions are extreme.[2-4]

In addition to reducing metabolic heat production, rest breaks allow opportunity for purposeful rehydration efforts with limited gastrointestinal distress or sport distraction (eg, continuing game play, tactics). A preplanned, individualized rehydration regimen is prudent for athletes when activity duration is long and large sweat rates are expected (> 1 L/h). Otherwise, athletes should be encouraged to drink slightly beyond thirst but not to discomfort during rest periods, limiting hyponatremia risk. During this time, diminished energy stores should be replenished in the form of carbohydrates, improving exercise performance during bouts of prolonged physical activity.

The use of cooling interventions, before or during sport, has recently grown as evidence builds supporting enhanced performance[5] and reduced risk of exertional heat illness. The benefit of intermittent body cooling during exercise is likely due to reducing the detrimental effects of hyperthermia on performance. However, wearing cooling garments or devices is not always feasible or practical during sport or occupational settings (firefighters, occupational workers, military). Instituting intermittent rest breaks during exercise enables the use of cooling interventions. Several portable and practical cooling modalities have been invented; however, only a few have sought valid independent scientific investigation, with few demonstrating valuable cooling effects.

It is recommended that individuals undergoing prolonged and/or intense bouts of physical activity include rest periods even if fluids are available during exercise. This recommendation is of particular importance during exercise in oppressively hot, humid conditions. Rest periods allow vital recovery time to (1) reduce metabolic heat gain, (2) dissipate accumulated thermal load, (3) clear metabolic byproducts that limit exercise, (4) restore energy reserves, (5) improve fluid and food intake, and (6) provide cooling interventions which reduce the risk of exertional heat injury and improve physical performance. Table 9-1 summarizes the benefits achieved when incorporating rest periods into physical activity.

Table 9-1

Benefits of Rest Periods During Exercise

	Improve Performance	Reduce Hyperthermia
Reduce metabolic heat production	↑	↑↑
Dissipate accumulated heat gain	↑↑	↑↑
Clear metabolic by-products	↑↑	↔
Food consumption	↑	↔
Fluid consumption	↑	↑
Cooling modalities	↑	↑↑

↑ indicates an increase in the benefit, ↑↑ indicates a substantial increase in the benefit, ↔ indicates no appreciable benefit.

References

1. Lopez RM, Casa DJ, Jensen KA, et al. Examining the influence of hydration status on physiological responses and running speed during trail running in the heat with controlled exercise intensity. *J Strength Cond Res.* 2011;25(11):2944-2954.
2. Casa DJ, et al. National Athletic Trainers' Association position statement: exertional heat illnesses. *J Athl Train.* 2015;50.
3. Armstrong LE, Casa DJ, Millard-Stafford M, Moran DS, Pyne SW, Roberts WO. American College of Sports Medicine position stand. Exertional heat illness during training and competition. *Med Sci Sports Exerc.* 2007;39(3):556-572.
4. Maresh CM, Sokmen B, Armstrong LE, et al. Repetitive box lifting performance is impaired in a hot environment: implications for altered work-rest cycles. *J Occup Environ Hyg.* 2014;11(7):460-468.
5. Ranalli GF, DeMartini JK, Casa DJ, McDermott BP, Armstrong LE, Maresh CM. Effect of body cooling on subsequent aerobic and anaerobic exercise performance: a systematic review. *J Strength Cond Res.* 2010;24(12):3488-3496.

Do Exertional Heat Illnesses Occur in a Continuum (ie, Heat Cramps → Heat Exhaustion → Exertional Heat Stroke) or Can They Occur Independently of Each Other?

Rebecca M. Lopez, PhD, ATC, CSCS

Before we knew much about exertional heat illnesses (EHI), there were quite a few misconceptions about them. Research in military and athletic settings has really enlightened us with information about these conditions. Unfortunately, there is often still a gap between the available knowledge base and clinical practice. It is imperative for athletic trainers to have a full understanding of the etiology of EHI in order to better prevent, recognize, and treat these conditions (Table 10-1).

One of the more common misconceptions regarding EHI is that they occur in a continuum. For instance, some may believe that one EHI is a warning sign for the next. In fact, it was often taught that if an athlete experienced exertional heat stroke (EHS), it was because the athlete had experienced heat exhaustion and was not treated properly. However, the actual definition of heat exhaustion is the inability to continue exercise in the heat due to cardiovascular insufficiency,[1,2] often as a result of dehydration, sodium loss, or energy depletion.[3] Therefore, by definition alone, it is not likely that someone who is unable to continue exercising will then succumb to EHS. When including heat cramps and heat syncope into the

Lopez RM, ed. *Quick Questions in Heat-Related Illness and Hydration: Expert Advice in Sports Medicine* (pp 49-52).

Table 10-1
Key Points in Recognizing Exertional Heat Illnesses

- Each EHI is a stand-alone condition that can occur independently of the others.
- An individual may collapse from EHS without warning or the presence of heat exhaustion.
- A victim of EHS will often still be sweating, since he or she was just exercising in the heat.
- The initial presentation for various heat illnesses is similar; an accurate recognition is the key to a positive outcome.

discussion, it can further cloud the issue. It is also not likely that someone suffering from heat cramps will progress to heat exhaustion, then EHS if not treated. Heat syncope, defined as fainting in a hot environment,[1] is caused by hypotension and will not likely progress to other heat illnesses either. Confusion in this area exists because some of the initial signs and symptoms for heat illnesses are similar. The following section gives examples and provides rationale to illustrate that EHI do not occur in a continuum.

EHS can have a sudden onset. When marathon runners collapse from EHS during a race, they often do so without warning. Survivors of EHS often mention that they experienced some signs, such as headache, dizziness, fatigue, and feeling hot but were still able to continue running for a few miles before actually collapsing and becoming unconscious.[3,4] In cases that involve the medical tent staff, however, a marathon runner may suddenly collapse near the end of the race (mile marker 20 to 26) with no previous warning and a body temperature well above 105°F. Therefore, these events demonstrate that heat exhaustion is not necessarily a precursor to EHS. With heat exhaustion, the initial signs and symptoms may be more obvious (pallor, feeling faint, vomiting). With these signs and symptoms, the individual is often unable to continue exercising due to dehydration, fatigue, and cardiovascular insufficiency. It is not clear then how heat exhaustion can lead to EHS if exercise ceases. It is important to note, however, that many of the signs and symptoms of both heat exhaustion and EHS are quite similar.

Real-life cases of EHS where an individual collapses without warning during exercise tell us that heat exhaustion does not *have* to be present in order for EHS to occur. But does this mean that it is impossible for someone who experiences heat exhaustion to continue to exercise and potentially experience EHS? This is difficult to ascertain. Consider the following scenario. Suppose a football player is experiencing heat exhaustion while running sprints at the end of practice. The athlete begins to vomit, exhibits pallor, is weak, and claims to feel lightheaded. At this point it would be quite difficult for him to actually be able to continue sprints. However, if he were to be pushed to continue running by coaches or teammates—despite signs and symptoms of heat stress—it is possible that his body temperature may continue to rise due to an increased intensity, dehydration, etc. In this case, one cannot say that it is impossible, given the presence of various factors that may lead to EHS (exercise intensity, dehydration, poor physical fitness, body composition, among others).

However, what normally happens in the case of heat exhaustion is that in the presence of an athletic trainer or other health care professional, the athlete stops exercising and removes his helmet and shoulder pads, and steps are taken to cool him down (taking him to a shaded or cooler area, applying ice towels, and administering oral fluids, if possible). In cases of heat exhaustion, these small steps often result in significant improvements in a short amount of time. If this athlete were to not receive treatment but were to stay down on one knee and not take off his equipment but not continue exercising either, it is unlikely that his body temperature would increase to the point of EHS, *particularly* if his body temperature was not dangerously elevated to begin with. Suppose now that this same football player experienced heat exhaustion during a morning practice and is now returning for the afternoon practice on the same day. It is actually very possible that experiencing heat exhaustion the previous day or even the same day may predispose this athlete to EHS if he has not adequately recovered.

It is important for clinicians to note that heat exhaustion is often a diagnosis of exclusion. Once it is evident that an individual is experiencing some form of heat stress, it is up to the clinician to determine the condition and severity. It is often difficult to distinguish heat exhaustion from EHS without measuring the patient's rectal temperature.[3] An individual may present with what seems like heat exhaustion and then experience a rapid decline in CNS function—aggressive behavior, going in and out of consciousness, and often becoming completely unresponsive—along with a dangerously elevated core temperature (> 104°F). Although some may believe that the presence of heat exhaustion is what led to EHS, it is more likely that it was EHS all along.

Conclusion

Knowing the causes and signs and symptoms of the different EHI will aid the clinician in making the correct diagnosis and determining the best course of action. It is not likely that the presence of a heat illness will lead to another more severe condition. However, an initial accurate recognition of the condition along with delivery of the appropriate treatment can ensure a successful outcome.

References

1. Armstrong LE. *Exertional Heat Illness*. Champaign, IL: Human Kinetics; 2003.
2. Casa et al. Inter-Association Task Force on Exertional Heat Illnesses consensus statement. *NATA News*. 2003;June:329-343.
3. Casa DJ, et al. National Athletic Trainers' Association position statement: exertional heat illnesses. *J Athl Train*. 2015;50.
4. Stearns RL, Casa DJ, O'Connor FG, Lopez RM. Heat illness—two marathon runners: a comparative case study. Free communications oral presentation. American College of Sports Medicine Annual Symposium, May 2011.

QUESTION 11

IS IT POSSIBLE TO PREVENT DEATH FROM EXERTIONAL HEAT STROKE?

Yuri Hosokawa, MAT, ATC, LAT and
Douglas J. Casa, PhD, ATC, FACSM, FNATA

Yes. Death from exertional heat stroke (EHS) within the confines of an organized physical activity is 100% preventable. Fatalities from EHS are preventable with immediate recognition and rapid cooling with appropriate methods.[1] Previously documented fatal cases of EHS have occurred as a result of common errors in the recognition, treatment, and/or characteristics of the workout session (Table 11-1). In many cases, the cause of death is multifaceted, with a cascade of events observed in fatal cases.[2] However, it is also important to emphasize that with appropriate plans for EHS management and organizational effort to lessen the predisposing risk factors, those factors are avoidable in most instances.

The ultimate reason for EHS death is multiorgan failure, which occurs when the heat stress surpasses the threshold for the body to maintain homeostasis and dissipate excess heat through the thermoregulatory response. The multiorgan failure may include failure of the cerebrum, adrenal glands, lungs, myocardium, diaphragm, spleen, kidneys, liver, intestines, and vascular system.[2] These damages and potential fatalities can be prevented through rapid, on-site cooling of the victim,

Lopez RM, ed. *Quick Questions in Heat-Related Illness and Hydration: Expert Advice in Sports Medicine* (pp 53-56).
© 2015 Taylor & Francis Group.

Table 11-1
Common Errors Observed in Fatal Exertional Heat Stroke Cases
• Lack of and/or inaccurate temperature assessment • Disregarding the environmental conditions (eg, WBGT) • No care provided for EHS • Delayed treatment • Inefficient cooling method • Not following "cool first, transport second" • Incomplete recovery from previous EHS or illness • Disregarding the fitness level • No authority to self-pace the workload

which minimizes the damage to organs and cells of the body.[3] The goal is to rapidly cool in order to lower the victim's core body temperature below 104°F (40°C) within the first 30 minutes (prior to transport to the hospital).[1]

Exertional Heat Stroke in the Military

It is critical for clinicians, coaches, and athletes to understand the predisposing factors of EHS to properly prevent and recognize such factors as they arise. Rav-Acha et al documented 6 fatal EHS cases in the Israeli Defense Forces in which the victims were all classified as heat-tolerant individuals before the incidents.[2] Each of the documented cases involved a unique cascade of events that contributed to the fatality. For example, in 3 of the 6 cases, the victims had an underlying illness that hindered them from participating in their regular training sessions the day before the EHS. The content of the training during which the soldiers experienced EHS differed by cases; however, many similarities were observed, such as exercise that occurred during the hottest hours of the day with a high wet bulb globe temperature (WBGT) and solar radiation, training that was unmatched to physical fitness, improper work-to-rest ratios, and improper rehydration regimens. In addition, improper diagnosis and treatment of EHS were documented in many cases, and absence of proper medical triage was reported in all 6 cases.

In the Marine Corps Recruit Depot at Parris Island, a total of 252 heat stroke victims were treated in a 15-year period, all of which were treated with ice-water immersion with no fatalities.[3] In this series of cases, most of the 252 EHS victims received rapid cooling within 20 minutes of collapse. Furthermore, the reports of EHS victims at Parris Island (N=25), which included the documentation for the presence of organ complications, and the cases from Beaufort Naval Hospital (N = 39) revealed no organ failures and fatalities when the victims were rapidly treated with water immersion.[3]

Exertional Heat Stroke in the Athletic Setting

Grundstein et al[4] analyzed 58 cases of fatal hyperthermia incidents in American football that were documented by the National Center for Catastrophic Injury Research. Linemen and athletes with high body mass index were identified as high-risk athletes, representing a large and disproportionate percentage of these deaths. On the days when the fatalities occurred, environmental stress related to the heat index was underestimated when compared with WBGT guidelines. Over 60% of the deaths occurred in conditions where the practice should have been canceled if the WBGT guidelines had been followed.

In contrast, there are cases of nonfatal EHS documented from the Falmouth Road Race (Falmouth, MA).[5] The Falmouth Road Race is a 7-mile (11.26-km) road race that is held on the second Sunday of August every year. The level of race participants ranges from novice to elite runners, and there have been a total of 361 cases of exertional heat illness reported in the race, including 274 cases of EHS and 87 cases of heat exhaustion during the span of 18 years (1984, 1989, 1992 to 1994, 1996 to 1998, and 2003 to 2011).[5] When a runner's rectal temperature is above 104°F (40°C) and there is central nervous dysfunction, the runner is diagnosed with EHS and immediately transferred to a cold-water immersion tub for rapid cooling. The immediate recognition with accurate assessment of core body temperature via rectal thermometer and rapid on-site cooling of the body using cold-water immersion at the Falmouth Road Race medical tent follows the gold standard of care for an EHS victim. There was 100% survival from EHS among all the victims who were brought to the medical tent, from the years included in this study and also during the years following.

Solutions

The common errors summarized in Table 11-1 are all manageable through institutional effort to provide appropriate on-site care that follows the best current practice. All personnel involved in an organized sport (eg, athletic trainers, coaches, athletic directors, league administrators, students, parents) need to be aware and informed and to act upon the best practices available. Appropriate knowledge and education on topics regarding the management and care of EHS should encourage the involved personnel to have an emergency action plan and to have a rectal thermometer, WBGT device, and cold-water immersion tub readily available on site. Sharing a consensus on appropriate management and care of EHS among all personnel will also assist in organizing safe practices and athletic events.

Conclusion

Recognizing common errors reported in the past literature and screening for the risk of those errors at individual settings (eg, high school football team practice, road race, off-site cross-country meet) become imperative in preventing EHS deaths. It is also important to note that when EHS is verified by measuring a rectal temperature above 104°F (40°C) and by the presence of central nervous system dysfunction, clinicians must immerse the victim in a cold-water tub while continuously circulating the water.[5] The early recognition and appropriate cooling method play a substantial role in maximizing the victim's chance of survival.[1,3] Clinicians must follow the best evidence-based practice available and tailor the prevention procedures accordingly to fit the unique circumstances of each setting. It is not an overstatement to say that fatality from EHS is 100% preventable in organized settings when trained medical personnel are present and implement appropriate plans for immediate recognition and rapid cooling.

References

1. Casa DJ, Armstrong LE, Kenny GP, O'Connor FG, Huggins RA. Exertional heat stroke: new concepts regarding cause and care. *Curr Sports Med Rep.* 2012;11(3):115-123.
2. Rav-Acha M, Hadad E, Epstein Y, Heled Y, Moran DS. Fatal exertional heat stroke: a case series. *Am J Med Sci.* 2004;328(2):84-87.
3. Costrini A. Emergency treatment of exertional heatstroke and comparison of whole body cooling techniques. *Med Sci Sports Exerc.* 1990;22(1):15-18.
4. Grundstein AJ, Ramseyer C, Zhao F, et al. A retrospective analysis of American football hyperthermia deaths in the United States. *Int J Biometeorol.* 2012;56(1):11-20.
5. DeMartini JK, Casa DJ, Belval L, et al. Effectiveness of cold water immersion in the treatment of exertional heat stroke at the Falmouth Road Race. *Med Sci Sports Exerc.* 2014;June 30. Epub ahead of print.

SECTION II

DIAGNOSIS

WHAT CRITERIA ARE USED TO DIFFERENTIATE BETWEEN HEAT EXHAUSTION AND EXERTIONAL HEAT STROKE?

Rebecca M. Lopez, PhD, ATC, CSCS and
Candi D. Ashley, PhD

On a summer day in the southeast region of the United States, it is the second football practice of the day, and the team is in full football gear. You are the athletic trainer, and 1 hour into the second practice you notice that one of the linebackers begins to stagger, vomits, and then drops to one knee. What is going on? Differentiating between exertional heat exhaustion and exertional heat stroke (EHS) can mean the difference between life and death. Exertional heat exhaustion is the most common exertional heat illness in athletes, soldiers, and civilians,[1] while EHS is one of the top 3 causes of sudden death in athletes.[2] The health implications of these 2 heat illnesses result in a tough situation for a clinician trying to decipher whether an athlete is experiencing heat exhaustion or EHS.

Heat exhaustion is characterized by the inability to continue to exercise in the heat.[3] Heat exhaustion can be caused by fluid loss or electrolyte loss, often referred to as water-depletion heat exhaustion or salt-depletion heat exhaustion, respectively.[1] The reduction in exercise capacity ultimately occurs because of the inability of the cardiovascular system to meet the circulatory demands of the thermoregulatory

Lopez RM, ed. *Quick Questions in Heat-Related Illness and Hydration: Expert Advice in Sports Medicine* (pp 59-63).
© 2015 Taylor & Francis Group.

Table 12-1

Differentiating Between Heat Exhaustion and Exertional Heat Stroke

Heat Exhaustion		Exertional Heat Stroke
Recognition		
• Temperature < 104°F (40°C) • Mild CNS dysfunction (weakness, fatigue, faint) • **Vomiting** • **Hot skin and sweating** • **Unable to exercise**	← similar →	• Temperature > 104°F (40°C) • Obvious CNS dysfunction with possible lucid intervals • **Vomiting** • **Hot skin and sweating** • **Unable to exercise**
Treatment		
• **Remove extra clothing and equipment** • Move to shaded area • Oral rehydration, if possible • Elevate feet • Ice-cold towels	← similar →	• **Remove extra clothing and equipment** • Cold-water immersion (35 to 59°F) for 10 to 15 minutes or until temperature drops to 102°F (39°C)

*Bold text depicts symptoms and treatment goals that are similar for both heat exhaustion and EHS.

system, muscular system, and cutaneous blood flow to continue exercise and maintain a normal body temperature during exercise in the heat.

EHS, on the other hand, is a condition resulting from a dangerously elevated body temperature resulting from an increased metabolic heat production or a reduced heat dissipation capacity. The causes of EHS are multifactorial and can include improper work-to-rest ratios, fever, physical fitness unmatched to exercise demands, lack of acclimatization, clothing that insulates and/or inhibits the evaporation of sweat, and a hot and humid environment.[3]

Deciphering the difference between heat exhaustion and EHS can be challenging for a clinician, as the signs and symptoms can be similar (Table 12-1). Death from EHS is preventable with proper recognition and treatment; therefore, it is imperative for clinicians to make this distinction. When an athlete collapses in the heat, the physical presentation of both conditions can be similar. Athletes with either condition may present with staggering or collapse, hot skin, pallor, nausea, and vomiting. It is not uncommon for an athlete experiencing heat exhaustion to

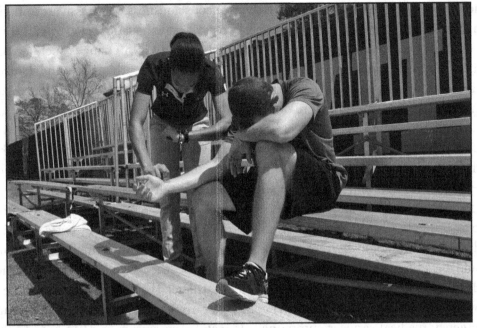

Figure 12-1. Initial presentation of heat exhaustion.

also feel faint (Figure 12-1) and have changes in skin color. It is a myth that a person experiencing EHS will not be sweating; it is imperative that clinicians *not* use the presence of sweat on the skin as a means to rule out EHS. The 2 main criteria for diagnosing EHS are (1) central nervous system (CNS) dysfunction presented as loss of consciousness, irritability, confusion, and/or irrational behavior, and (2) an elevated body temperature (rectal temperature > 104°F).[4]

Although the most effective treatment for these conditions may vary, the initial steps in treatment are similar. The cessation of exercise, removal of excess clothing (socks, shoes) and equipment (helmet, shoulder pads), and moving the athlete to a cooler area in conjunction with fluids (oral, if tolerable) are often an effective treatment for heat exhaustion (see Table 12-1). In a football player, for example, simply removing the helmet and shoulder pads, moving the athlete to a shaded, cooler area, and administering oral fluids will result in dramatic improvements in thermoregulation in a short amount of time. Placing an ice-cold towel over the head and shoulders also helps with the recovery. If the athlete is feeling faint, putting him or her in a supine position and elevating his or her feet may also result in improvements with heat exhaustion. The athlete will begin to regain normal skin color, not feel faint, and claim to feel better after these simple measures are taken. However, no more than 10 minutes should be spent in deciding if it is EHS or heat exhaustion.

These immediate improvements noted with effective treatment of heat exhaustion will not occur in cases of EHS. Although someone experiencing EHS may appear lucid for a short time, the athlete's condition will often worsen, with CNS function quickly deteriorating to either unconsciousness, aggressive/combative behavior, or acting out of sorts. In cases of severe heat exhaustion, however, it is not uncommon for the athlete to feel faint and have mild CNS changes such as mild confusion. In this scenario, distinguishing between heat exhaustion and EHS is paramount. The most important criterion in differentiating between heat exhaustion and EHS is a valid measure of core body temperature (gastrointestinal or rectal).[4] It is not unusual for an athlete exercising in the heat to have an elevated core body temperature (ie, > 98.6°F); however, a rectal temperature of > 104°F together with CNS dysfunction should lead the clinician to a diagnosis of EHS—a medical emergency. Recognition of these conditions can be a diagnosis of exclusion.

If EHS is suspected and the athlete collapses and is unconscious, CNS dysfunction is immediately evident. After ruling out a cardiac condition, extra clothing and equipment should be removed and a rectal (or gastrointestinal) temperature should be obtained. The clinician should not use the "wait and see" approach with an unconscious or obviously obtunded athlete. If the rectal temperature is above 104°F, whole body cooling via cold-water immersion should be initiated and emergency medical services summoned. If rectal temperature is < 104°F and other differential diagnoses have been ruled out (eg, exertional sickling, concussion), heat exhaustion should be diagnosed. In this case, rotating ice-cold towels, dousing with cold water, or other alternate cooling methods in conjunction with rehydration should be continued. If a rectal temperature is unavailable and a heat illness is suspected, cold-water immersion should be initiated.

Using rectal temperature in cases of severe heat exhaustion allows the clinician to adequately diagnose and provide the appropriate treatment. In one case at a local high school, the athletic trainer (JK, oral communication) was dealing with a case of severe heat exhaustion that she initially began treating as heat exhaustion (dousing with cold water, oral fluids). The athlete's condition began to deteriorate, and she obtained a rectal temperature (101.5°F). In this case, it is unknown what the athlete's initial temperature was; however, the athletic trainer was then confident that she needed to stay the course and continue with her treatment.

If a valid diagnosis is not made on the field and the athlete is transported to the hospital, there is a possibility that the patient's temperature will not be taken immediately. If the patient is suffering from EHS and his or her temperature has been elevated above 104°F for an extended time (> 45 to 60 min), the chances of survival are low.[4,5] A sustained elevated temperature experienced with EHS will likely result in elevated serum enzymes, multisystem organ failure, and potentially death. With heat exhaustion, however, blood tests will reveal normal enzyme levels, and treatment with intravenous fluids will often result in a complete recovery.[1] This demonstrates the importance of being able to differentiate between these

2 conditions on the field, in order to deliver the appropriate treatment *prior* to transport to the hospital.

Conclusion

When an athlete presents with signs and symptoms of heat illness, it is imperative for the clinician to be able to distinguish between heat exhaustion and EHS—a medical emergency. Those suffering from heat exhaustion will often show improvements with 10 to 15 minutes of treatment (removing clothing, oral rehydration, cooling methods); however, an athlete experiencing EHS will show a decline in CNS functioning and display a rectal temperature greater than 104°F. Using these diagnostic tools is the key to making an accurate diagnosis, giving the appropriate treatment, and ensuring survival.

References

1. Armstrong LE, Lopez RM. Return to exercise training after heat exhaustion. *J Sport Rehab.* 2007;16(3):182-189.
2. Casa DJ, Anderson SA, Baker L, et al. The Inter-Association Task Force for sudden death in collegiate conditioning sessions: best practice recommendations. *J Athl Train.* 2012;47(4):477-480.
3. Casa DJ, et al. National Athletic Trainers' Association position statement: exertional heat illnesses. *J Athl Train.* 2015;50.
4. Casa DJ, Guskiewicz KM, Anderson SA, et al. National Athletic Trainers' Association position statement: preventing sudden death in sports. *J Athl Train.* 2012;47(1):96-118.
5. Armstrong LE, Casa DJ, Millard-Stafford M, et al. American College of Sports Medicine position stand: exertional heat illness during training and competition. *Med Sci Sports Exerc.* 2007;39(3):556-572.

WHAT TEMPERATURE DEVICES ARE VALID WHEN MEASURING INTERNAL BODY TEMPERATURE IN AN EXERCISING INDIVIDUAL?

Rebecca L. Stearns, PhD, ATC and Julie K. DeMartini, PhD, ATC

Obtaining an accurate body temperature for an exercising individual can be a very important, life-saving step. In the case of exertional heat stroke (EHS), where diagnosis includes a body temperature that is equal to or greater than 104°F (40°C) with associated central nervous system dysfunction,[1] obtaining an accurate body temperature is the only objective measure that can differentiate EHS from a wide variety of other conditions. Differential diagnoses may include other conditions that may also have central nervous system dysfunction.[1] These can range from non–life-threatening to life-threatening conditions, such as heat exhaustion, exertional sickling, hyponatremia, concussion, cardiac event, etc. A body temperature of 104°F or greater is the one symptom that separates EHS from these other conditions and, in the medical field, can help to quickly diagnose or rule out this condition when time is crucial for life-saving treatment.

Examples of devices and body sites that have been used to assess body temperature include esophageal, pulmonary artery, oral, aural (tympanic), temporal artery, gastrointestinal, forehead, rectal, and axillary. The main concern when measuring

Lopez RM, ed. *Quick Questions in Heat-Related Illness and Hydration: Expert Advice in Sports Medicine* (pp 65-69).
© 2015 Taylor & Francis Group.

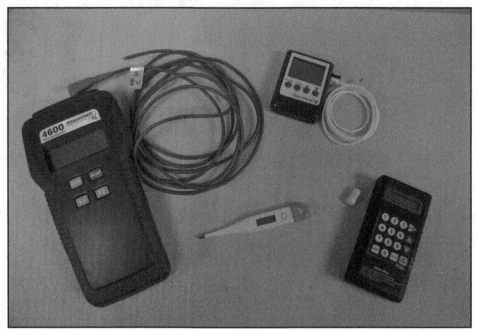

Figure 13-1. Various temperature monitoring devices: clockwise from left: YSI rectal thermometer with probe, DataTherm rectal thermometer with probe, HQ CorTemp receiver and sensor (gastrointestinal temperature), and regular thermometer that can be used rectally.

body temperature in an exercising individual is that the skin and blood flow responses are very different from those measured in a resting individual. In addition, the environment, skin sweat, recently ingested fluids, and skin temperature could all potentially influence the accuracy of a body temperature measurement, depending on the site of that measurement. A consistent line of research has established that rectal temperature is the only acute and accurate method of obtaining body temperature for an exercising individual, likely because it is resistant to these external influences (sweat, skin blood flow, sun, etc).[2,3]

Two recent research studies[2,3] examined the validity of a myriad of body temperature devices. These studies compared oral (expensive and inexpensive devices), aural (expensive and inexpensive devices), temporal (via 2 measurement techniques), axillary, forehead sticker, and gastrointestinal temperature with rectal temperature during exercise both indoors[3] and outside.[2] These studies both confirmed that the only valid device (measuring within 0.5°F of rectal temperature) during exercise in the heat was gastrointestinal temperature. These studies also noted that in some cases devices possessed high correlations and reliability, though they were not valid body temperature measures. Lastly, researchers found no correction factor for any device, as the measures obtained did not have a predictable factor by which it could be accurately compared to rectal temperature. Figure 13-1 illustrates various temperature devices that can be used to accurately measure rectal or gastrointestinal temperature.

The only devices that have been consistently demonstrated to provide an accurate body temperature assessment for an exercising individual measure rectal, esophageal, pulmonary artery, and gastrointestinal temperatures.[2-5] These are generally considered the gold standards given that a thermometer in these locations will measure blood that is circulating within the heart, brain, and deep organs of the body, all vital to a person's health and physiological functioning. Even these methods come with their own advantages and disadvantages (Table 13-1). Pulmonary artery assessment is very invasive and takes time and precision to properly place the thermistor in addition to compliance on the part of the patient. Taking an esophageal reading is similar, in that a thermistor must be inserted through the nasal cavity and down the back of the throat, which also requires compliance on the part of the patient. Although these 2 methods may be appropriate in research settings, they are not practical in a clinical setting. Gastrointestinal and rectal temperatures are the only 2 remaining accurate methods. While gastrointestinal temperature has been proven valid in comparison with rectal temperature assessment, the telemetric pill must be ingested a minimum of 5 hours before an accurate reading can be collected. (The pill needs to be in the intestines and have passed through the stomach for accuracy.) Therefore, the only location where a device can obtain an acute and valid body temperature measure for an individual who has been exercising is rectal.

Recently, a study examined the use of body temperature devices during exercise in the cold. This study also used rectal temperature as the gold standard to compare aural, axillary, forehead, gastrointestinal, oral, and temporal readings. Every device (with the exception of the gastrointestinal telemetric pill) measured temperatures significantly lower than rectal temperature; therefore rectal and gastrointestinal temperatures are also valid assessment tools during exercise in the cold.[5]

While rectal temperature is the gold standard for obtaining a body temperature in an exercising individual for immediate medical diagnosis, it is also important to consider the location of any valid thermometer in relation to the measure obtained. For example, rectal temperature has been reported to have a lag in response time compared with esophageal or pulmonary artery temperature, which is likely due to the location of the rectal thermometer (in a deep body cavity versus a highly vascularized cavity of the body).[2] This is one of the main reasons why it has been established that EHS patients should be removed from cold-water immersion tubs when their rectal temperature reaches 102°F, because their body temperature will continue to drop and because of the slight lag in the temperature assessed at the rectum compared with the esophageal or pulmonary artery location. This is why it is important to remember that even with the use of a validated body temperature assessment, the location of the measure should be a consideration when interpreting body temperature.

Table 13-1

Comparison of Various Temperature Monitoring Devices

Temperature Device	Advantages	Disadvantages	Valid Measurement in Individuals Exercising in the Heat?
Esophageal	True measurement of core body temperature	Invasive; not practical in a clinical (nonlaboratory) setting	Yes
Pulmonary artery	True measurement of core body temperature	Invasive; not practical in a clinical (nonlaboratory) setting	Yes
Oral	Easy to use; inexpensive	Influenced by outside variables (ie, eating, drinking, air temperature, breathing, swallowing)	No
Aural (tympanic)	Easy to use; inexpensive	Not true tympanic membrane temperature	No
Temporal artery	Easy to use	Measures only skin temperature; variable due to sweat production, skin temperature, ambient temperature, etc	No
Axillary	Easy to use; inexpensive	Uses sheltered skin temperature for measurement	No
Forehead sticker	Easy to use	Measures only skin temperature, variable due to sweat production, skin temperature, ambient temperature, solar radiation, etc	No

(continued)

Table 13-1 (continued)

Comparison of Various Temperature Monitoring Devices

Temperature Device	Advantages	Disadvantages	Valid Measurement in Individuals Exercising in the Heat?
Rectal	Gold standard of body temperature measurement for athletes exercising in the heat; can be inexpensive	Can be expensive; invasive; requires skill of medical professional	Yes
Gastrointestinal (ingestible thermistor)	Easy to use; can monitor core body temperature during exercise; can monitor several athletes at once	Can be expensive for prolonged monitoring of a large team; each pill is good for only 1 use (~1 day); pill must be ingested several hours before time of reading	Yes

Overall, rectal temperature has been shown to be the only quick, valid, and effective method of obtaining body temperature in an exercising individual. Using an invalid device not only will provide an inaccurate measure but could affect proper medical diagnosis and treatment. Medical professionals who wish to obtain body temperature in cases of suspected EHS or other exercise-associated collapse should only do so by means of rectal temperature assessment.

References

1. Casa DJ, Guskiewicz KM, Anderson SA, et al. National Athletic Trainers' Association position statement: preventing sudden death in sports. *J Athl Train*. 2012;47(1):96-118.
2. Casa D, Becker S, Ganio M, et al. Validity of devices that assess body temperature during outdoor exercise in the heat. *J Athl Train*. 2007;42(3):333-342.
3. Ganio MS, Brown CM, Casa DJ, et al. Validity and reliability of devices that assess body temperature during indoor exercise in the heat. *J Athl Train*. 2009;44(2):124-135.
4. Pearson J, Ganio MS, Seifert T, et al. Pulmonary artery and intestinal temperature during heat stress and cooling. *Med Sci Sports Exerc*. 2012;44(5):857-862.
5. Bagley JR, Judelson DA, Spiering BA, et al. Validity of field expedient devices to assess core temperature during exercise in the cold. *Aviat Space Environ Med*. 2011;82(12):1098-1103.

CAN SKIN TEMPERATURE BE USED TO ASSESS AN ATHLETE'S BODY TEMPERATURE WHEN EXERCISING?

Luke N. Belval, ATC, CSCS and
Lesley W. Vandermark, MS, ATC, PES

Skin temperature may appear to be an easy alternative to some of the more invasive methods of "core" or deep-body temperature assessment; however, several obstacles exist that prevent this from being a viable option. Since it tracks very poorly with rectal temperature, skin temperature is not a valid measure of body temperature in exercising individuals.[1] Skin temperature can be influenced by a variety of factors both from within the body and from the external environment. Furthermore, the methods for assessment of skin temperature are variable and costly, and can be impractical.

Skin temperature does play an important role in thermoregulation; the temperature gradient between the skin and the deep-body tissues is the principal method to dissipate heat created during exercise in stressful environments.[2] As skin temperature increases, the gradient that allows for heat to flow from deep tissues and exercising muscle decreases and can lead to dangerous increases in core body temperature. Figures 14-1 and 14-2 demonstrate the 2 contrasting scenarios that may occur when exercising in the heat. During compensable heat stress (see Figure

Lopez RM, ed. *Quick Questions in Heat-Related Illness and Hydration: Expert Advice in Sports Medicine* (pp 71-74).

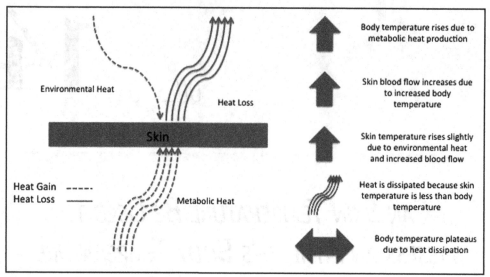

Figure 14-1. Exercising in the heat (compensable).

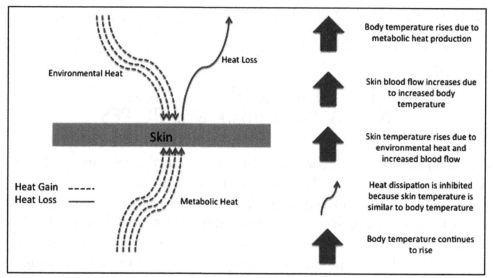

Figure 14-2. Exercising in the heat (uncompensable).

14-1), the external environment does not place an excessive heat load on the skin surface that would prevent the body from dissipating heat from an increased skin blood flow. Alternatively, when environmental conditions prevent or overwhelm heat dissipation (see Figure 14-2), the skin temperature will rise and the temperature gradient necessary for cooling diminishes. Therefore, it can be seen that only in the situation of thermoregulatory failure would skin temperature likely be equivalent to body temperature.

The largest internal determinant of skin temperature during exercise is the amount of blood flow to the skin.[2] As demonstrated by Sawka et al, even small decreases in the skin temperature to core temperature gradient can create very large increases in skin blood flow.[2] During exercise, skin blood flow is increased to aid in dissipating heat created by exercising muscles. However, when skin blood flow is unable to unload this heat through evaporation, convection, conduction, or radiation, skin temperature will concurrently rise and may ultimately contribute to thermoregulatory failure.

Environmental conditions also have a large influence on skin temperature during exercise, which presents an additional challenge to the clinician. In fact, the skin temperature responses of an individual are influenced by the environment more than any type of homeostatic thermoregulatory control.[2] The ambient temperature, solar radiation, and humidity of a given environment all have effects on the skin temperature.[3]

Ambient temperature and solar radiation directly heat the skin and, when the skin temperature meets or exceeds the surrounding environment, heat dissipation becomes less efficient. Solar radiation can also affect skin temperature when an individual becomes sunburned.[3]

During exercise, when the body is able to fully dissipate heat, the primary method of heat dissipation is evaporation of sweat. This requires that the water vapor pressure (ie, humidity) of the surrounding area be able to absorb the fluid from sweat. However, high humidity decreases this water vapor pressure gradient, which does not allow for sweat to evaporate off the skin surface. This greatly reduces the efficiency of sweating, as it prevents evaporation and may be uncomfortable for exercising individuals. Since evaporation is inhibited, the heat contained in the sweat remains on the skin surface, which can lead to increases in skin temperature.

Clothing and equipment can also cause variance in skin temperature, as it may aid or impede thermoregulation. Clothing worn while exercising may create a microenvironment that does not allow sweat to evaporate from the skin surface.[4] This phenomenon was the impetus for wicking materials that draw moisture away from the skin and may help keep an individual cool. When an individual is wearing heavy equipment, such as football pads or military gear (nuclear, biological, chemical gear), creating uncompensable heat stress, heating of the skin becomes even more dangerous. This extra clothing and equipment can create an additional insulating effect that traps heat on the skin's surface. Athletes can have very different skin temperatures in the heat based on the clothes and equipment they wear, confounding the relationship between skin temperature and body temperature. An athlete wearing full football pads and long sleeves may have a very different skin temperature at a practice in 20°C (68°F) than if he or she were in short sleeves and no pads.

The current standard for assessing skin temperature is through the use of weighted formulas.[1] These formulas use point measurements taken from 4 to 14 anatomical sites across the body to be weighted and calculate an overall mean skin temperature. This can be performed using either contact thermistors (eg, iButtons) or a noncontact infrared thermometer. Commonly used equations can be found in Choi et al[5] and ISO 9886.[1] Another emerging method of skin temperature assessment is the use of thermal imaging with infrared cameras; however, cameras typically cost in excess of $10,000, and methods for analysis vary widely.

Skin temperature plays a large role in how an individual is able to cope with heat stress during exercise. However, due to confounding factors both internally and externally, skin temperature assessment alone lacks clinical validity and relevance. Clinically, a "true" mean skin temperature is less relevant than understanding the interplay between the environment, core temperature, and skin surface temperature. Understanding that an individual wearing equipment and exercising in a hot, humid environment will not only feel hotter but also have his or her body temperature rise quicker because of high skin temperatures is crucial to preventing and treating exertional heat illnesses. For that reason, it is more important and likely more practical to determine risk of heat illness by wet bulb globe temperature monitoring during exercise.

In the case of a suspected exertional heat illness, accurate body temperature assessment should be performed. Any temperature reading that measures skin temperature should not be used alone. When used in conjunction with rectal or gastrointestinal temperature, skin temperature may provide additional information on the amount of heat stress an individual is undergoing. Ultimately, the clinician should rely on the validated methods of body temperature assessment (ie, rectal or gastrointestinal temperature) and the monitoring of environmental conditions in the prevention and management of exercise in the heat.

References

1. ISO 9886. *Ergonomics: evaluation of thermal strain by physiological measurements.* 2004:1-21.
2. Sawka MN, Cheuvront SN, Kenefick RW. High skin temperature and hypohydration impairs aerobic performance. *Exper Physiol.* 2012;97(3):327-332.
3. Casa DJ. Exercise in the heat: I. Fundamentals of thermal physiology, performance implications, and dehydration. *J Athl Train.* 1999;34(3):246.
4. Gavin TP. Clothing and thermoregulation during exercise. *Sports Med.* 2003;33(13):941-947.
5. Choi JK, Miki K, Sagawa S, Shiraki K. Evaluation of mean skin temperature formulas by infrared thermography. *Int J Biometeorol.* 1997;41(2):68-75.

WHAT ARE THE STEPS TO CORRECTLY USE A RECTAL PROBE IN ORDER TO DIAGNOSE AND MONITOR A POSSIBLE CASE OF EXERTIONAL HEAT STROKE?

Lesley W. Vandermark, MS, ATC, PES and
William M. Adams, MS, ATC

Rectal thermometry is the gold standard tool for recognition of exertional heat stroke (EHS). It is the most valid and reliable tool for assessing body temperature and is the only valid method to use on exercising individuals. Rectal thermometry should be included in emergency action plans as part of the protocol for recognizing and treating EHS.[1] An elevated rectal temperature > 104°F (40°C) and the presence of central nervous system (CNS) dysfunction are the key diagnostic criteria to determine the presence of EHS.[1,2] Of the various methods that are available to assess temperature, only rectal temperature and gastrointestinal temperature have been found to be valid and reliable measures of temperature in exercising individuals.[1,2] Rectal thermometry is considered the gold standard because it measures the temperature of the rectum, which is deep in the body in a similar location to several vital organs. Measuring rectal temperature is part of the curriculum in all accredited athletic training education programs, and athletic trainers are expected to perform it when EHS is suspected.[3] Rectal temperature should be used to

Lopez RM, ed. *Quick Questions in Heat-Related Illness and Hydration: Expert Advice in Sports Medicine* (pp 75-78).
© 2015 Taylor & Francis Group.

diagnose a life-threatening condition. It should not be used if signs and symptoms of CNS dysfunction are not present in an athlete. Health care providers should use discretion and careful judgment before using rectal thermometry.

Rectal thermometry should be part of EHS protocols in your emergency action plan, provided that the venue has the appropriate equipment. Commonly in some settings (eg, high schools), parents or administrators may be hesitant to allow medical staff to use a rectal thermometer. However, this commonly stems from a lack of understanding of the necessity of the device, the essential purpose for which it is used, and the exact protocol for use, which protects the patient. Administrators may require additional information about rectal thermometry. They should be educated about EHS and the potential risks and benefits of using rectal thermometry as a means of diagnosis. A resource from the National Athletic Trainers' Association is the "Heat Illness Treatment Authorization Form," which provides information and space for authorization of use of rectal temperature in the diagnosis and treatment of EHS.[4]

Obtaining a rectal temperature is easy, fast, and accurate. Table 15-1 refers to the steps a health care professional should take to appropriately use a rectal thermometer to assess temperature.[5] Many concerns about using a rectal probe surround the issues of privacy and invasiveness. In terms of privacy, it is the duty of the health care professional to use the best tools for the task at hand.[3] If a female patient were to be in cardiac arrest, one would never think twice about exposing her chest to apply defibrillator pads. This concept should also be applied to diagnosing EHS. While the privacy of the patient is important, his or her safety is paramount. To help protect privacy, the patient should be draped with a towel or sheet so that his or her private area is not exposed.[5] It would also be prudent to move the athlete to a somewhat private area. When working with young athletes, another adult, preferably a coach or administrator, should be present with the health care provider during the probe insertion. Having another adult who understands the emergency protocols of the venue may be helpful if questions arise about the situation. Because the athlete is experiencing CNS dysfunction, he or she may be unconscious, confused, combative, or disoriented. Be sure to talk to the patient if he or she is conscious; explain what you are doing and that it is important. Inserting the probe may take some help from others, including fellow athletes and coaches, to help keep the athlete calm. They can help the patient relax as much as possible while the probe is inserted efficiently, so that treatment follows quickly.

Although there are different types of thermometers that can be used rectally with a collapsed athlete, the use of a flexible rectal probe with a thermometer that reads to at least 110°F (43.3°C) is recommended in the athletic setting. These probes are long, flexible thermistors, which are inserted 10 cm beyond the anal sphincter. The health care provider should wear gloves and be sure to clean the

Table 15-1

Twelve Steps for Using a Rectal Thermometer on a Collapsed Athlete

1. Remove the athlete from the playing field, if appropriate, to a shaded area.
   a. Use a tent, locker room/athletic training room, or area under a tree.
2. Drape the patient appropriately with a towel or sheet, if possible.
3. Position the patient side-lying with top knee and hip flexed forward.
4. Make sure the probe is cleaned with isopropyl alcohol.
5. Lubricate the rectal probe, if necessary.
6. Make sure the probe is plugged into the thermometer.
7. Turn the thermometer on.
8. Insert the probe 10 cm past the anal sphincter.
   a. To prepare, measure this ahead of time and draw a line on the probe.
9. If you meet resistance while inserting, stop and remove, then try again.
10. If flexible probe, leave the probe in for the duration of treatment to monitor temperature.
    a. If rigid, reinsert probe every 5 minutes during treatment to monitor temperature.
11. After treatment, remove the probe gently.
12. Clean the probe with sterilization solution or other protein-removing soap.

Adapted from the Korey Stringer Institute website, http://ksi.uconn.edu/information/athletic-trainers/heat-considerations.

probe with an alcohol swab prior to insertion. The thermistor is small, less than 1/8th of an inch in diameter. Flexible probes may be submerged and remain in place during treatment, which allows temperature to be continuously monitored. Rigid probes or standard thermometers may be used rectally; however, these may not remain in place during treatment. The biggest drawback with using a standard thermometer is that it could not be submerged in water during cold-water immersion. However, if a rigid probe is all that the health care provider has during treatment, the athlete should have the probe inserted periodically to assess temperature during treatment and make decisions about when to stop treatment.[1,2] This should occur approximately every 5 minutes, but it should be noted that removal from the cooling modality might cause the necessary cooling time to increase slightly, therefore putting the patient at increased risk.[5]

If possible, the probe should remain inserted in the patient during treatment so that the athlete's temperature may be continuously monitored.[1,2] As a note, due to rectal temperature lag, the effects of the cooling treatment the athlete is receiving may not be apparent for the first 5 minutes or so. After the first few minutes, rectal temperature will rapidly decline at a rate consistent with the cooling modality being applied. The faster the cooling rate, the more likely the athlete is to survive the EHS without sequelae. The advantage to keeping the probe in place during treatment is that the health care provider can see the temperature decline and make decisions about when to stop cooling the athlete. The athlete should be removed from the cooling modality when rectal temperature reaches 102°F (39°C).[1,2]

The final step in using a rectal thermometer is cleaning the probe. Once the athlete has reached a safe temperature (102°F or below) and has finished cooling, the probe can be gently removed from the patient. The probe should be sterilized so that it can be reused. Sterilization using a solution takes approximately 10 hours of being immersed in the solution. This can be done in any container as long as it can be covered and protected against circulating air. Other soapy products that remove proteins also sufficiently clean the probe. The probe can then be rinsed, dried, and packed again for future use.[5]

References

1. Armstrong LE, Casa DJ, Millard-Stafford M, et al. American College of Sports Medicine position stand: exertional heat illness during training and competition. *Med Sci Sports Exerc.* 2007; 39(3):556-572.
2. Binkley HM, Beckett J, Casa DJ, Kleiner DM, Plummer PE. National Athletic Trainers' Association position statement: exertional heat illnesses. *J Athl Train.* 2002;37(3):329-343.
3. Mazerolle SM, Scruggs IC, Casa DJ, et al. Current knowledge, attitudes, and practices of certified athletic trainers regarding recognition and treatment of exertional heat stroke. *J Athl Train.* 2010;45(2):170-180.
4. National Athletic Trainers' Association position statements page. National Athletic Trainers' Association website. http://www.nata.org/sites/default/files/Heat-Stroke-Treatment-Authorization-Form_0.pdf. Accessed May 22, 2013.
5. Korey Stringer Institute Heat Considerations for Athletic Trainers Page. Korey Stringer Institute website. http://ksi.uconn.edu/information/athletic-trainers/heat-considerations. Accessed May 22, 2013.

HOW DOES ONE DIFFERENTIATE BETWEEN AN EXERTIONAL HEAT ILLNESS AND AN EXERTIONAL SICKLING EVENT?

Robert C. Oh, MD, MPH and Francis G. O'Connor, MD, MPH

Why Is It Important to Know About Sickle Cell Trait?

Sickle cell trait (SCT) is common, with millions of affected individuals. In the United States it is found in 8% of Blacks, 0.5% of Hispanics, and 0.2% of Whites.[1] SCT is an inheritable condition that is generally benign and of little consequence to the affected individual. Two parents who carry SCT, however, have the potential to give birth to a child with sickle cell disease, which can be an extremely challenging medical condition for the affected individual. Accordingly, screening for SCT is historically important, in particular with regard to preconception counseling. Recently, however, deaths among athletes associated with SCT, in particular collegiate football players, have been well documented in the medical literature and the media. Once thought to be inconsequential in the sports setting, SCT has been shown to have a 22 times increased risk for sudden death among Black Division 1 National Collegiate Athletic Association (NCAA) football players.[2] In 2010, the

Lopez RM, ed. *Quick Questions in Heat-Related Illness and Hydration: Expert Advice in Sports Medicine* (pp 79-83).
© 2015 Taylor & Francis Group.

NCAA initiated a policy requiring documentation of sickle cell status or having the athlete sign a waiver forgoing testing.

Exertional sickling events, also known as exercise collapse associated with sickle cell trait (ECAST) events, have been described most commonly among American football players and among the military, particularly in new recruits. Most cases have occurred prior to the start of the football season, or during recruit training, and have nearly always been associated with intense conditioning training, such as sprinting. The trigger appears to be related to intensity of exercise as the critical first event leading to fulminant rhabdomyolysis. However, both dehydration and heat can be cofactors, and the exact mechanism of these events remains speculative.

Why Does ECAST Cause Sudden Death?

The mechanism of how an ECAST event can lead to a sudden death event is debated. Several authors postulate that ECAST events are the result of an exertional sickling event that leads to fulminant rhabdomyolysis with associated metabolic consequences—a term labeled *explosive rhabdomyolysis*. Intense exercise, sometimes with heat stress and dehydration, may set off a cascade of hypoxemia, lactic acidosis, and red cell dehydration—leading to acute red cell sickling, inflammation, vascular occlusion, and eventual exertional collapse. The ensuing explosive muscle breakdown triggers rapid release of potassium, causing hyperkalemia and, hence, the risk for fatal cardiac arrhythmia.

How Does ECAST Present on the Field?

ECAST may be the first sign of impending explosive rhabdomyolysis.[3] Overall, clinical reports of exertional sickling are strikingly similar—initial collapse, associated with intense exercise, typically sprinting at or near maximal exertion. Pain can be severe, intense, and cramp like; however, there are no visible signs of cramping (eg, muscle twitching). Therefore, pain is generally out of proportion to exam, and the athlete is unable to walk due to profound muscle weakness. Importantly, the athlete is conscious and early on does not have major mental status changes. This conscious collapse, while not universally present in all ECAST events, can be a critical discriminator from other forms of exercise-associated collapse. The ECAST event can have various outcomes, including resolution, continued leg pain that can be a harbinger of a fulminant rhabdomyolysis, or decompensation into cardiopulmonary arrest.

Commonality to Exertional Heat Illness

Exertional collapse in a hot, humid environment may lead the clinician to assume heat illness. In fact, one US Army study reported that 22 of 30 cases of ECAST were associated with exertional heat illness (EHI).[1] Additionally, a large-scale study completed but never published by the US Army demonstrated that limiting work and heat exposure and enforcing adherence to water hydration guidelines practically eliminated sudden death related to SCT. However, the role of heat stress and dehydration and its association with exertional sickling remain controversial. A closer look at the reported cases shows no seasonal predilection, which argues against heat being an independent risk factor for exertional sickling. Also, in the 15 most recent cases of exertional sickling in the military, there was no evidence of exertional heat stroke (EHS; E. Eichner, personal communication). Most cases involved elevated body temperature, but this was usually less than 102°F, and this mild hyperthermia may have represented normal temperature excursions related to exercise and not a true heat illness. The common thread of EHS and exertional sickling is exertional collapse associated with end-organ damage. After that, the similarities end, and the management diverges widely. Therefore, recognition of each entity is critical to the survival of the athlete (Table 16-1).

Differentiating From Exertional Heat Illness

The term *exertional heat illness* generally encompasses heat cramps, heat exhaustion, and heat stroke. If an athlete's sickle cell status is known, any exertional collapse associated with exercise should heighten the potential of exertional sickling. Also, a critical discriminator is that EHS victims present immediately with acute confusion and change in mental status, while in exertional sickling the athlete is commonly conversant at first. Second, body core temperature is generally less than 104°F in exertional sickling, whereas core temperature is 104°F or greater in an EHS victim. Core temperature elevation occurs commonly with exercise but is generally less than 104°F. If there are no mental status changes and temperature is not above 104°F, then it is critical to ascertain for muscle pain and weakness. In exertional sickling, the muscles remain soft and flaccid, as opposed to the painful involuntary muscular contractions associated with heat cramps. Additionally, muscle cramps are usually associated with long, endurance exercise, as opposed to the brief and intense duration of exercise associated with exertional sickling. In heat exhaustion, there generally is mild muscle pain and exhaustion, which responds well to rest, shade, and oral or intravenous hydration. Any associated muscle pain and weakness out of proportion to exam should be treated by having oxygen administered, an intravenous line started, and immediate transport of the athlete

Table 16-1

Differentiating Exertional Heat Illness From Exertional Sickling

	Muscle Cramps	Heat Exhaustion	Exertional Heat Stroke	Exertional Sickling
Presentation	Extreme pain and hobbling	Exhaustion, no collapse	Exertional collapse	Exertional collapse-slumps
Mental status	Normal	Normal	Acute changes, confusion	Conscious and conversant; can rapidly progress to coma
Core temperature	Normal	< 104°F	≥ 104°F	< 104°F
Associated risk factors	Heat, previous history of heat cramps	Exertion in heat	Heat, medications, dehydration	Sickle cell trait, preseason conditioning
Duration of exercise	Prolonged duration	Prolonged duration	Prolonged heat exposure	Brief, intense duration
Muscles	Painful, tense, spasms	Mild pain and weakness	Mild pain	Profound weakness > pain, soft, and flaccid more than pain
Treatment	Massage, stretches, oral hydration	Rest, shade, oral or IV hydration	Rapid, immediate cooling	Early recognition, oxygen and immediate transport

to the hospital.[4] If sickle cell status is known, then clear communication to expect fulminant rhabdomyolysis and a potential need for dialysis should be relayed to the receiving hospital team.

Additionally, it is important to recognize that it is possible for an athlete with SCT to have an EHS event, which may in turn be complicated by exertional sickling. When in doubt, the provider needs to move emergently with early cooling and then forward the patient to the emergency department with the receiving facility aware of the potential for the metabolic crisis of exertional sickling. While this chapter has sought to identify "clinical clues" to assist the provider in differentiating these 2 life-threatening illnesses, each case is unique, and urgency and judgment are required of the prudent clinician.

Prevention Strategies

Limiting maximal or near maximal intense training early in the season may help reduce the risk for ECAST. A slower paced training and conditioning program that allows for longer rest periods and recovery, generally at the athlete's own pace, may help reduce ECAST events.[4] Although the relationship of heat stress and dehydration remain unclear, ensuring hydration during times of heat load and stress may mitigate the cascade of events leading to ECAST. In addition, if training at altitude, the athlete should be monitored closely, training should be modified, and oxygen immediately available. The role of universal screening, despite the NCAA's recent requirement, remains controversial.[3]

Conclusion

Early recognition of exertional sickling and differentiating it from EHI is critical, since management is quite divergent and may be life saving. EHI can be recognized by assessment of mental status, core temperature, and examination for muscle cramps. On the other hand, exertional collapse in an athlete with SCT who is mentally clear and has profound muscle weakness and pain out of proportion to exam should be treated as a medical emergency, and the athlete should be transported immediately to a higher level of care.

References

1. Eichner ER. Sickle cell considerations in athletes. *Clin Sports Med*. 2011;30(3):537-549.
2. Harmon KG, Drezner JA, Klossner D, Asif IM. Sickle cell trait associated with a RR of death of 37 times in national collegiate athletic association football athletes: a database with 2 million athlete-years as the denominator. *Br J Sports Med*. 2012;46(5):325-330.
3. O'Connor FG, Bergeron MF, Cantrell J, et al. ACSM and CHAMP summit on sickle cell trait: mitigating risks for warfighters and athletes. *Med Sci Sports Exerc*. 2012;44(11):2045-2056.
4. Casa DJ, Guskiewicz KM, Anderson SA, et al. National Athletic Trainers' Association position statement: preventing sudden death in sports. *J Athl Train*. 2012;47(1):96-118.

SECTION III

EMERGENCY MANAGEMENT AND TREATMENT

WHAT IS THE BEST PRACTICE FOR THE TREATMENT OF EXERTIONAL HEAT ILLNESSES (HEAT CRAMPS, HEAT SYNCOPE, HEAT EXHAUSTION, AND EXERTIONAL HEAT STROKE)?

Nicholas D. Peterkin, MD; Joseph S. Atkin, MD; and
Eric E. Coris, MD

Heat-related illness in athletics is a common condition. The National Center for Catastrophic Sports Injury Research reports a total of 52 deaths in football players due to exertional heat stroke (EHS) from 1995 to 2012.[1] Although heat injury can be fatal, the majority of cases are not and are preventable. Hot and humid conditions are the single most critical predisposing risk factor.[2] As with many medical conditions, the best treatment is prevention, which can be accomplished by using a good preparticipation exam, evaluating for predisposing conditions or medications, ensuring proper hydration, and observing weather conditions. During sports events, monitoring exercising athletes for signs of disease and having a good emergency plan in place for possible EHS is critical for protecting athletes. Heat illness may present as mild heat edema or heat cramps to more severe heat syncope, heat exhaustion, or heat stroke. Early recognition based on signs and symptoms should prompt immediate action to limit progression of injury (Table 17-1).

Exertion-associated muscle cramps (EAMC) are defined as painful muscle spasms following prolonged strenuous exercise, often in the heat.[3] Treatment is

Lopez RM, ed. *Quick Questions in Heat-Related Illness and Hydration: Expert Advice in Sports Medicine* (pp 87-91).

Table 17-1

Heat Illness Symptoms, Signs, and Treatment

	Symptoms	Signs	Treatment
Exertional associated muscle cramps	Painful muscle cramps	Palpable muscular spasm	Stretch, ice, massage, oral fluids
Heat syncope	Syncope	Loss of consciousness	Rest, supine with feet up, monitor vital signs
Exertional heat exhaustion	Fatigue, inability to continue exercise, mild confusion, nausea, vomiting, syncope, "chills" of head and neck	Hypotension, orthostasis, elevated core temperature (up to 40.5°C), syncope	ABCs, cool, rest, monitor temp/VS, oral fluids
Exertional heat stroke	Pronounced mental status changes, fatigue, nausea, vomiting, syncope	Elevated core temp > 40.5°C, hypotension, tachycardia, tachypnea, syncope, possible cessation of sweating, coma, DIC, ARF	ABCs, cool urgently, call emergency services, monitor VS, IVF if available.

Abbreviations: ABC, airway, breathing, circulation; ARF, acute renal failure; DIC, disseminated intravascular coagulation; IVF, intravenous fluids; VS, vital signs.

Adapted from Coris EE, Ramirez AM, Van Durme DJ. Heat illness in athletes: the dangerous combination of heat, humidity, and exercise. *Sports Med.* 2004;34(1):9-16.

aimed at stopping the cramps and limiting progression. Immediate treatment of EAMC is with a prolonged stretch of the affected muscle at full length. Muscle cramps can be debilitating and extremely painful. Allow the athlete to rest out of play while you manage the cramps. If possible, cool the affected muscle with ice packs or a towel soaked in cold water. Gently stretch the muscle group past neutral as tolerated to try to "break" the spasm. Replace sweat-induced fluid and sodium loss. This is ideally accomplished by oral rehydration, such as with a commercial sports drink, or these can be made with 1/8 to 1/4 teaspoon of table salt added to 300 to 500 mL fluids.[3] Replacement can also be in the form of salt tablets taken with 300 to 500 mL of fluid or salty snacks.[3] With severe cramping, oral replacement is difficult and may require parenteral administration. Intravenous normal saline provides rapid relief, usually with 1 to 2 L; however, this requires establishing intravenous access and monitoring clinically, typically with a physician present. This may be too time consuming for immediate return to play, but possibly necessary if cramping is severe. Refractory cramping can be treated with benzodiazepines intravenously; however, these require monitoring for sedation and exclude return to play that day.[3] Intravenous benzodiazepines would also require the presence of a physician to monitor the patient. Once cramping has resolved, the athlete can return to play as tolerated but is at risk for recurrent cramping. Muscle soreness may limit participation, and the athlete may need one or more days to recover. Severe cramping may be a warning sign of impending heat exhaustion[4] and should be monitored closely.

Heat syncope is a transient loss of consciousness in an athlete, with abrupt cessation of exertion or sudden elevating postural changes in the heat.[4] The syncope is due to orthostatic hypotension and inadequate blood flow to the brain.[4,5] The diagnosis is clinical.

Treatment of heat syncope relies on recognizing athletes and areas (such as at the finish chute of an endurance event) most at risk. Try to keep the participants from standing still immediately after exertion. Continuing movement will help venous blood return to the heart by using the muscle pump of the contracting leg muscles. If the individual is near fainting or has fainted, lay him or her supine and elevate the legs above heart level to assist in venous return.[4,5] Monitor vital signs, including rectal temperature, if EHS is considered. Replace fluids, ideally by mouth, if dehydration is a factor. This clinical scenario is usually short lived, and the goal is to avoid the dangers of falling. Ensure that the patient is safe when getting up to avoid the dangers of fainting/falling again. Prevent the athlete from rising too quickly from a supine or sitting position.

Exertional heat exhaustion is defined as the inability to continue exercise during heavy exertion in the heat and may include physical collapse.[3,5] Treatment of exertional heat exhaustion involves cooling, rest, and fluid rehydration. The athlete should be moved to a cool or shaded place for closer evaluation and treatment. Cooling therapy improves medical status. Monitor vital signs. If the rectal temperature cannot be checked, empiric cooling therapy, as described in the next section, should be considered.[3] Lay the athlete down, with legs elevated to aid blood flow return. Oral fluids are preferred, but for the athlete who cannot tolerate oral ingestion or has more severe dehydration, intravenous fluids with normal saline can lead to a rapid improvement from heat exhaustion.[3] Monitor the patient until he or she is alert with clinically stable vital signs. The athlete can then be discharged from the event or sidelines with instructions for continued rest and rehydration. Return to play that day is not advised. If athletes do not improve despite these efforts, or

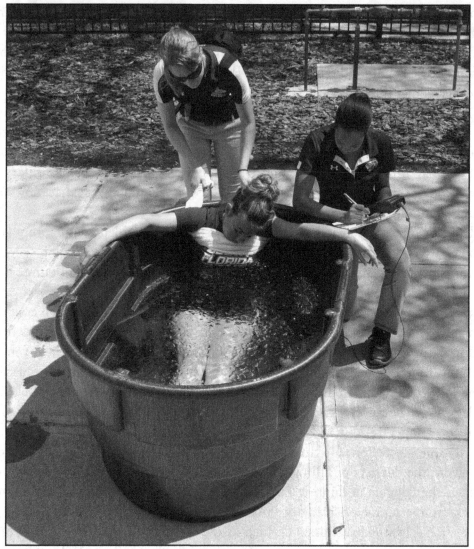

Figure 17-1. An athlete immersed in a cold-water tub, attended by 2 athletic trainers.

exhibit a progressive clouding of consciousness, they should be transported to an emergency facility for further medical management.

EHS is defined as hyperthermia with a core temperature greater than 40°C and associated central nervous system disturbances and multiple organ failure.[3] Any individual with possible EHS should have his or her rectal temperature measured.[5]

Treatment of suspected or confirmed EHS involves removal of any clothing or gear that limits heat dissipation and immediately cooling the whole body via cold-water immersion (Figure 17-1). EHS is a true medical emergency, as it can be fatal, and any delay in cooling can worsen the prognosis. Cold-water immersion provides the fastest cooling rate with lowest morbidity and mortality.[3] Any event where EHS has a high likelihood of occurring should have cold-water tubs available. If there are no means of immersing the athlete in cold water, use ice packs and towels/sheets dipped in cold water and apply them to the neck, groin, axilla, and extremities. Constantly rotate the ice packs or towels every 2 minutes for more rapid cooling. Monitor the blood pressure, rectal temperature, and heart rate continuously. Intravenous normal saline will maintain intravascular volume and ensure good renal blood flow. If no intravenous fluids are available, oral rehydration should be used if the patient is coherent and able to swallow. Ensure that the individual is cooled until the rectal temperature is safely below 40°C,[3] other vital signs are normal, and mental status is normal. If the patient continues to decline despite cooling efforts, immediately transfer him or her to an emergency facility for further management. Those whose conditions are recognized early and who are cooled instantly often show a complete return of vital signs to baseline. Emergency medical personnel should always be contacted in cases of suspected EHS.

Heat-related illnesses are very common. They range from heat cramps to potentially fatal EHS. There are several modifiable risks, such as length and intensity of heat exposure. These can be optimized by ensuring good hydration and, when possible, coordinating heat acclimatization. Although there are several signs and symptoms of exertional heat exhaustion and stroke, they are not specific and require early recognition, treatment, and monitoring. Outcomes are generally good with early and appropriate intervention.[5] Most important is educating athletes, coaches, and athletic training staff about the dangers of exercise in the heat.[5] When managing events, ensure that the appropriate medical staff and equipment[5] is on hand to monitor patients, estimate core temperatures with a rectal thermometer, and rapidly cool and rehydrate athletes.

References

1. Kucera KL, Klossner D, Colgate B, Cantu RC. Annual survey of football injury research, 1931-2013. National Center for Catastrophic Sports Injury Research, University of North Carolina at Chapel Hill, March 2014.
2. Marshall SW. Heat Injury in youth sport. *Br J Sports Med.* 2010;44:8-12.
3. American College of Sports Medicine, Armstrong LE, Casa DJ, et al. American College of Sports Medicine position stand. Exertional heat illness during training and competition. *Med Sci Sports Exerc.* 2007;39(3):556-572.
4. Coris EE, Ramirez AM, Van Durme DJ. Heat illness in athletes: the dangerous combination of heat, humidity, and exercise. *Sports Med.* 2004;34(1):9-16.
5. Casa DJ, et al. National Athletic Trainers' Association position statement: exertional heat illnesses. *J Athl Train.* 2015;50.

If You Do Not Have a Rectal Probe for the Proper Assessment of Body Temperature, What Should You Do if You Suspect an Athlete Has Exertional Heat Stroke?

Riana R. Pryor, MS, ATC and J. Luke Pryor, MS, ATC, CSCS

Medical professionals have the challenging task of performing a differential diagnosis when an individual collapses during physical activity. Many signs (including collapse) and symptoms of life-threatening conditions are similar among illnesses, causing difficulty differentiating between them.[1] Examples of conditions that can result in collapse include, but are not limited to, exertional heat stroke (EHS), cardiac conditions, traumatic brain injury, exertional hyponatremia, exertional sickling, hypoglycemia, and respiratory distress. All of these conditions cause athletes to exhibit central nervous system (CNS) dysfunction, fatigue, and staggering, among other symptoms.

Medical providers can use a decision algorithm to determine treatment options when EHS is suspected. An example of an appropriate algorithm is displayed in Figure 18-1. Specific details about the situation are often used to try to narrow down the possible causes for a collapsed athlete. The timing of the patient's collapse (ie, end of a race or intense practice), environmental conditions (ie, hot or humid environment), clothing (ie, heavy clothing or equipment), and visual reason

Lopez RM, ed. *Quick Questions in Heat-Related Illness and Hydration: Expert Advice in Sports Medicine* (pp 93-96).

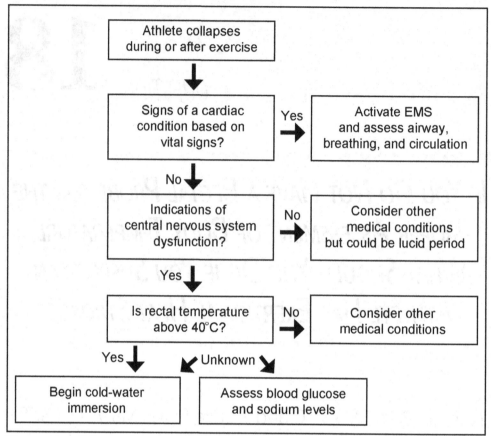

Figure 18-1. Differential diagnosis of a collapsed athlete.

for collapse (eg, no collision indicating head injury) are all details to consider indications of EHS and should cause medical providers to consider this condition.

When an athlete collapses, it is necessary to decide what the various differential diagnoses are and if EHS should be included as a possibility. Cardiac conditions should be ruled out first because of the imminent danger to the athlete. Once it is concluded by taking vital signs that the person is still breathing and has circulation, CNS function should then be assessed. During this time, look for key signs of CNS dysfunction, including disorientation, confusion, aggression, irrational behavior, headache, nausea, dizziness, and weakness. These signs and symptoms are indicative of EHS, but are also indicative of other life-threatening conditions, such as traumatic brain injury, hypoglycemia, and hyponatremia. Brain injury should be considered if the athlete collided with another athlete, object, or the ground.

If the patient is responsive, a brief medical history should be taken to gather information about previous history of collapse, sickle cell trait status, allergies, and concomitant complaints. If the person is responsive but is exhibiting signs of CNS dysfunction (eg, confusion, aggression, unaware of surroundings), a rectal temperature should be taken. Similarly, if the athlete is not responsive, rectal temperature should be used as a definitive tool to diagnose EHS. If this equipment is not available upon patient collapse, it is imperative that no other body temperature measurements are used in its place due to the low reliability and validity of other temperature sites with exercising individuals.[2]

Even if rectal temperature is not available, athletes should be suspected of having EHS if the medical provider can answer "yes" to some of the following questions: (1) Does the person have an altered level of consciousness? (2) Is the person suffering from convulsions? (3) Did the person collapse during intense exercise in the heat? and (4) Have other causes of collapse been ruled out?[3] If "yes" is answered for Question 4 and at least one other question, the athlete should be moved to a shaded or indoor area, and all excess equipment and clothing should be removed prior to commencement of immediate cold-water immersion (CWI). If the athlete is conscious and has the ability to drink, fluid replacement should be encouraged. To rule out other conditions such as hypoglycemia or hyponatremia, a blood sample should be taken to analyze serum glucose and sodium, should necessary equipment be available. These measurements, however, should not delay CWI.

When rectal temperature is not available during CWI, the body temperature of the patient remains unknown during cooling. CWI studies suggest that the cooling rate using this modality varies based on water temperature, but this modality generally cools at a rate of $0.15°C$ to $0.35°C \cdot min^{-1}$ ($0.27°F$ to $0.63°F \cdot min^{-1}$).[4] After approximately 10 minutes of CWI, the body can cool $1.5°C$ to $3.5°C$. A typical EHS patient can have a rectal temperature of $40°C$ to $42°C$ ($104°F$ to $107.6°F$), and within 10 minutes the patient would cool to a rectal temperature below the critical temperature threshold ($40°C/104°F$) for cell damage. Therefore, when medical staff is unable to obtain rectal temperature during CWI, the patient should be kept in the water for approximately 10 minutes before being transferred to the hospital for further evaluation.

It is important to note that some EHS patients may begin with an extremely high body temperature (eg, $> 42°C/107.6°F$), and 10 minutes of cooling would not be sufficient to cool beyond the critical temperature threshold. Without an initial rectal temperature, these dangerously high body temperatures would not be known. Similarly, if the patient is cooled for too long, signs and symptoms of hypothermia (eg, shivering; white, ashen, or cyanotic skin color; goose bumps) can develop, in which case the patient should be removed from the water and rewarmed with blankets and a warm beverage. After the 10 minutes of cooling, the EMS team should transport the patient to the hospital for further evaluation.

One example of a misdiagnosed heat stroke case occurred in a military recruit who collapsed after participating in a 1-hour night march ($26°C/78.8°F$, 78% relative humidity).[5] The soldier presented to the medical clinic with delirious and aggressive behavior, hyperventilation, and bouts of vomiting. The physician misdiagnosed the soldier as having conversion disorder, a neurological condition without a definitive etiology instead of the correct diagnosis of EHS. Four hours after seeking initial medical treatment, the patient was comatose and taken to the hospital, where a rectal temperature of 39.6°C (103.3°F) was reported. The soldier died 24 hours later.

This is an excellent example of a case where the physician should have suspected that a patient was suffering from EHS; however, this was not on the list of differential diagnoses or EHS was mistakenly ruled out. The warm, humid environmental conditions in which the soldier exercised and the CNS dysfunction (ie, collapse, aggressive and delusional behavior) should have led the medical provider to consider EHS. Had the soldier been properly cooled via CWI (whether or not a rectal temperature had been taken), he would have likely survived.

The opposite scenario is also possible, during which the medical staff may assume the athlete is presenting with EHS but the athlete is actually experiencing a different condition. Medical staff should not immediately suspect EHS before ruling out other conditions such as exertional sickling, cardiac conditions, traumatic brain injury, or concussion. Events leading up to the condition (eg, hit to the head or body, high intensity exercise with short rest periods) and medical history (eg, presence of sickle cell trait, family history of cardiac conditions) need to be considered when completing a differential diagnosis of an athlete. The only way to know for certain that EHS is occurring is to obtain a rectal temperature.

Definitive determination of EHS relies primarily on rectal temperature and CNS dysfunction, although rectal temperature may not always be available. In the latter case, the timing and exercise conditions during which the individual collapses, environmental conditions, clothing worn, and previous medical history should be considered when suspecting EHS. Once cardiac and other conditions are ruled out, EHS should be suspected and aggressive CWI should be implemented for approximately 10 minutes to begin to lower elevated body temperature prior to possible transport to the hospital.

References

1. Casa DJ, Pagnotta KD, Pinkus D, Mazerolle SM. Should coaches be in charge of care for medical emergencies in high school sport? *Athl Train Sports Health Care.* 2009;1(4):144-146.
2. Pryor RR, Seitz JR, Morley J, et al. Estimating core temperature with external devices after exertional heat stress in thermal protective clothing. *Prehosp Emerg Care.* 2011;16(1):136-141.
3. Casa DJ, Armstrong LE. Exertional heatstroke: a medical emergency. In: Armstrong LE, ed. *Exertional Heat Illnesses.* Champaign, IL: Human Kinetics; 2003:29-56.
4. Casa DJ, McDermott BP, Lee EC, Yeargin SW, Armstrong LE, Maresh CM. Cold water immersion: the gold standard for exertional heatstroke treatment. *Exerc Sport Sci Rev.* 2007;35(3):141-149.
5. Heled Y, Rav-Acha M, Shani Y, Epstein Y, Moran DS. The "golden hour" for heatstroke treatment. *Mil Med.* 2004;169(3):184-186.

How Should a Clinician Deal With a Combative Exertional Heat Stroke Victim?

Douglas J. Casa, PhD, ATC, FACSM, FNATA;
Luke N. Belval, ATC, CSCS; and
Rebecca M. Lopez, PhD, ATC, CSCS

It is ironic that unconscious exertional heat stroke (EHS) patients are often considered the easiest to treat. In medical tent situations the staff may actually feel thankful for the calm, cooling, and comatose patient because many of the cooling tubs could be occupied by those experiencing severe central nervous system (CNS) dysfunction, ranging from mood changes to combativeness. Many examples exist of patients who become mortified when they are informed of behaviors that they exhibited during treatment. The lessons to be learned are many (Table 19-1), and we hope these case studies serve as valuable learning tools for medical professionals.

Lopez RM, ed. *Quick Questions in Heat-Related Illness and
Hydration: Expert Advice in Sports Medicine* (pp 97-103).
© 2015 Taylor & Francis Group.

Table 19-1
Lessons Learned

Preparation	1. Be prepared for a variety of scenarios; EHS patients can display a variety of behaviors.
	2. In the mass medical tent, extra security personnel are useful.
	3. In a college or high school setting, coaches or other athletes may need to assist with treatment.
	4. We encourage readers to volunteer at mass medical tents so that they can see EHS up close and be prepared for treatment in their work setting.
Recognition	1. EHS can cause severe CNS dysfunction.
	2. Symptoms include irrational behavior, combative behavior, speaking nonsense, complete unconsciousness, altered consciousness, convulsions, violence, screaming, bizarre noises, and extreme headaches.
	3. Some patients will not exhibit extreme CNS changes immediately; a lucid interval may exist. If an athlete has collapsed following intense exercise in the heat and cardiac conditions have been ruled out, assume EHS until proven otherwise (a prompt rectal temperature confirms or refutes EHS finding).
Treatment	1. Even in the face of obscure or combative behavior, it is vitally important to treat an athlete as quickly as possible. Time cannot be wasted rationalizing or debating with patients.

Case 1: I Will Take Consciousness With That Gatorade

Scenario: Summer road race.

Patient: A 40- to 49-year-old female found near postrace recovery/hydration area.

Initial Temperature: 107.2°F.

Behavior: Runner was found in fetal position. After looking up her race number, we found out she had finished 12 to 15 minutes earlier. She was transported to the medical tent.

Outcome: After 18 minutes of cold-water immersion her rectal temperature was 102°F; she survived without complication. She informed us that she felt hot after the race and sought out hydration (hence the recovery area), before she succumbed to the EHS.

Clinical Consideration: Hyperthermic athletes may appear fine immediately after exercise but later demonstrate CNS dysfunction. This "lucid interval" (evidenced here by the patient's efforts to get fluids postrace) can make diagnosis difficult and underscores the importance of continuously monitoring athletes.

Case 2: Drowning in the Tub

Scenario: Summer road race.

Patient: A 30- to 39-year-old male who collapsed just before finishing.

Initial Temperature: 107.8°F.

Behavior: This individual exhibited numerous unique behaviors while being cooled: (1) He asked for his wife to remove the rectal thermometer. (2) He asked for a specific brand of beer (while using profanities). (3) He said he would drown himself if we did not get him out of the tub (he was near 108°F). He then dropped to his knees against our resistance (with one hand on each side of the tub) and performed a countdown to put his head under water. He then submerged his head and repeated this for good measure. We then had enough staff to overcome his force and ensure he was lying down in the tub.

Outcome: The patient's rectal temperature was down to 102°F after 21 minutes, and he survived without complication. Once he regained normal CNS function, we explained everything to him, and he was shocked. His wife verified that we were telling the truth.

Clinical Consideration: When an EHS patient becomes combative, more personnel are needed. When caring for any patient with EHS, we suggest having individuals who are able to help even if they are coaches or other athletes.

Case 3: Make a Run for It

Scenario: Summer road race.

Patient: A 30- to 39-year-old male who collapsed just after the finish line.

Initial Temperature: 106.8°F.

Behavior: While we were cooling this patient, he overpowered the staff, got out of the tub, and made a run for the exit while screaming nonsense. An emergency medical technician tackled him in the aisle of the treatment area; we then brought him back to the immersion tub and used more people to restrain him while we continued cooling.

Outcome: His rectal temperature was lowered to 102°F after 18 minutes of cold-water immersion, and he survived without complication. We told him he needed to work on his speed.

Clinical Consideration: As in the case above, an athlete being treated for EHS can change from being calm to combative at any time. It is important to prepare for these changes in behavior in order to be able to continue treatment.[1]

Case 4: Biting and Holding

Scenario: East coast marathon.

Patient: A 20- to 29-year-old female who collapsed just before the finish line (approximately a 3:45 finisher).

Initial Temperature: 108.2°F.

Behavior: This patient had severe CNS dysfunction while we were cooling her. She was kicking, punching, and eventually bit a physician, removing a piece of forearm. Her boyfriend, who witnessed this, thought we were harming her, so he ran over and tried to get her out. Other medical personnel immediately restrained him.

Outcome: Her rectal temperature was lowered to 102°F after 17 minutes of cold-water immersion, and she survived without complication. Her boyfriend was removed from the area until the patient was discharged.

Clinical Consideration: EHS patients may believe the treatment saving them is actually harming them. Even when the patient is demonstrating severe CNS dysfunction, it is important to remain professional and inform the patient of what you are doing to him or her and why. It is also helpful to keep family members and friends away and, if possible, have someone explain the situation to them.[1]

Case 5: If I Wish Them Away

Scenario: East coast marathon.

Patient: A 30- to 39-year-old male who collapsed just after finishing. He was a 3:15 finisher.

Initial Temperature: 106.5°F.

Behavior: While this patient was being cooled, he pulled me (DJC) close to him and asked if I could make everyone leave so that only I could take care of his EHS. He said everyone was too loud and making him nervous. His temperature was 106.5°F, and he was going in and out of consciousness.

Outcome: His rectal temperature was brought down to 102°F after 16 minutes of cold-water immersion; he survived without complication.

Clinical Consideration: Many patients will drift in and out of consciousness and apparently be calm throughout their treatment. While they are easier to manage, continuously talking to this patient is important to assess how the treatment is progressing.[1]

Case 6: Altercation With the Authorities

Scenario: Summer road race.

Patient: A 40- to 49-year-old male was encountered near postrace recovery area.

Initial Temperature: Over 107°F.

Behavior: This runner was acting out of sorts and yelling at people. When a police officer went to talk to him and restrain him, the runner punched the officer. As the police tried to arrest him, a medical staff member thought he might be experiencing EHS and had them bring him to the medical tent instead.

Outcome: His rectal temperature was lowered to 102°F after 21 minutes of cold-water immersion, and he survived without complication. He was not arrested.

Clinical Consideration: EHS patients who are normally polite and reserved can quickly become aggressive and violent. In cases where you know the athlete, any departure from the norm in terms of mood or cognition can be a sign of EHS.

Case 7: Rectal Temperature Debate With a Lawyer

Scenario: East coast marathon.

Patient: A 30- to 39-year-old male (3:30 finisher) who collapsed just after finishing.

Initial Temperature: 107.8°F.

Behavior: The patient was relatively conscious when he arrived to the medical tent. When we explained that we needed to take a rectal temperature, he asked if we could assess temperature another way, such as oral or tympanic. We explained that those were not accurate in this situation. He continued to ask for options, and we told him we had none.

Outcome: With additional staff, we forcefully assessed his rectal temperature as he resisted. He became unconscious within 5 minutes. He was cooled with cold-water immersion for 21 minutes until his temperature reached 102°F. He survived without complication. We later explained everything to him in the medical tent. He was embarrassed and begged us not to tell his wife. We did not tell her.

Clinical Consideration: Because of the invasive nature of rectal thermometry, many patients will resist, even when they are experiencing CNS dysfunction. It is advisable to stay calm, professional, and insistent when encountering these patients.[2]

Case 8: Pizza Delivery at a Soccer Field

Scenario: Summer soccer camp, midafternoon of third day (second practice of the day).

Patient: A 16-year-old male who collapsed during sprint drills. He was next to a fence with a coach when the athletic trainer arrived.

Initial Temperature: Not measured.

Behavior: The athletic trainer took over care and realized the athlete had CNS dysfunction. The athlete continually asked when the pizza would be arriving. Aggressive cooling via cold-water immersion was initiated.

Outcome: The patient was cooled for 20 minutes and survived without complication. The pizza never arrived.

Clinical Consideration: Abnormal behavior may appear to be humorous on the surface; however, these clues should be taken in context during exercise in the heat.

Case 9: The Escape

Scenario: NCAA Division III baseball practice, first nontraditional season practice, ambient temperature in excess of 90°F.

Patient: An 18-year-old freshman baseball player.

Initial Temperature: Not taken.

Behavior: This patient collapsed during the fourth hour of a practice. He remained conscious and able to respond to questions. Coaches initially applied wet towels and called 911. When emergency medical services arrived they removed the towels and moved the patient to an ambulance. Once inside the ambulance the patient became combative saying, "Why would you try to give me money?" and declaring, "She is trying to kill me!" about a female emergency medical technician. He then attempted to escape the ambulance as it was moving. His transport was delayed until police and an additional emergency medical services crew could arrive to restrain him. No treatment was given until he was at the hospital (more than 15 min later).

Outcome: The athlete ended up being transported to more advanced care for emergency surgery. The player suffered brain injury as a result of this EHS and the delay in care; he has not been able to recover fully.

Clinical Consideration: This case illustrates that an EHS patient can become so combative that it is easy to overwhelm the medical staff responsible for treatment. Any delay in treatment can have profound effects on the outcome, and medical staff should be prepared to restrain patients if necessary.

References

1. Casa DJ, Guskiewicz KM, Anderson SA, et al. National Athletic Trainers' Association position statement: preventing sudden death in sports. *J Athl Train.* 2012;47(1):96-118.
2. Casa DJ, Almquist J, Anderson SA, et al. The Inter-Association Task Force for Preventing Sudden Death in Secondary School Athletics Programs: best practices recommendations. *J Athl Train.* 2013;48(4):546-553.

HOW DO YOU PREPARE FOR AND APPROPRIATELY IMPLEMENT THE USE OF COLD-WATER IMMERSION FOR THE EMERGENCY MANAGEMENT OF EXERTIONAL HEAT STROKE?

William M. Adams, MS, ATC and Riana R. Pryor, MS, ATC

Exertional heat stroke (EHS) is a medical emergency, and prompt, aggressive steps to cool the body below 40°C (104°F) within the first 30 minutes is critical in saving an athlete's life. Cold-water immersion (CWI) is the "gold standard" in treatment of EHS, as it provides the most efficient whole-body cooling to lower core body temperature.[1-4] In addition, CWI is an easy and inexpensive way to treat EHS because the equipment can quickly be set up on a daily basis, and only water, ice, and a tub (or something that can be filled with ice and water and large enough to fit the largest person on the team) are required.

Preparation

Before CWI can be successfully used to treat an athlete with EHS, the treating athletic trainer must be prepared for implementation. It is essential to have a detailed, site-specific (ie, football field, soccer field, on/off campus) emergency action plan that is rehearsed annually with all personnel who could be involved

Lopez RM, ed. *Quick Questions in Heat-Related Illness and Hydration: Expert Advice in Sports Medicine* (pp 105-109).
© 2015 Taylor & Francis Group.

with patient care. More specifically, the emergency action plan should clearly detail the steps to take when dealing with a suspected case of EHS and the mode of treating the athlete.[2,5]

In regard to preparing to use CWI, it is important have an area set up for CWI prior to practices and games. This can be accomplished by filling up a water tub about half full of water prior to the practice or athletic event. The water tub can be any make or model, but must be large enough to fit any athlete, from a cross-country runner to a football lineman. Next to the tub, have four 10-gallon coolers full of ice that can be used to create the ice-water bath. It is important not to dump the ice in the water at the beginning of practice because the ice will melt immediately (especially on a hot day) and the water temperature will not be cold enough to cool an athlete with EHS quickly.

Equipment Needed

The equipment needed to appropriately implement CWI is minimal and rather inexpensive. Below is a list of necessary items that are needed for CWI.

- *Water source*: The water source must be easily accessible with an accompanying hose to fill a tub with water.

- *Water tub*: It is essential to have some sort of tub to fill with water in order to implement CWI. These tubs can range anywhere from the popular 100- to 150-gallon Rubbermaid stock tanks (Figure 20-1), kiddie pools, or even a whirlpool in the athletic training room.

- *Ice coolers*: It is recommended to have about four 10-gallon coolers that can be used to store ice until it is needed to treat an athlete with EHS.

- *Ice*: An ample amount of ice is needed to cool the water down to maximize the amount of cooling the athlete is receiving. It is recommended that the water temperature should be around 50°F when treating an EHS athlete.

- *Sheet/towels*: A sheet or towels are needed to place under the arms of the athlete being treated to help keep the head above the water line. Also, towels can be used to help cool any exposed parts of the body that are not in the water.

- *Gloves*: Wearing gloves is a universal precaution and should be followed when treating an athlete with EHS.

Basics of Treatment

Once it is determined that an athlete is suffering from EHS (rectal temperature > 40°C and obvious CNS dysfunction), whole-body CWI must be initiated

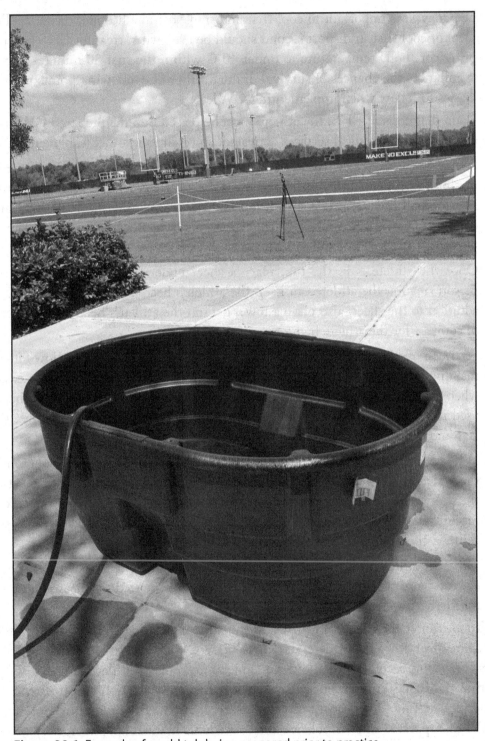

Figure 20-1. Example of a cold tub being prepared prior to practice.

immediately; it is important to cool first and transport to a hospital second.[1,2] The protocol of cool first, transport second should be used when treating EHS because lowering core body temperature to under 40°C within the first 30 minutes of collapse enhances the chances of survival dramatically.[2] The following points provide the basics to follow when implementing CWI.

- Upon diagnosis of EHS, the athlete must be placed into the prepared CWI tub and emergency medical services activated, since EHS is a medical emergency.

- It may be necessary to have a few people (4 to 6) assist the athletic trainer in placing the athlete in the tub, especially if the athlete is a larger individual (such as a football lineman). It is also important to remove any excess clothing and equipment (eg, shoes, socks, gloves, helmet, equipment, shoulder pads) prior to placement in the CWI tub to increase cooling capacity.

- Once the athlete is in the tub, place a sheet under the victim's arms so the person treating the athlete can keep the athlete's head above the water line. In addition to the sheet, also place a towel behind the athlete's head to add a level of comfort for the athlete being treated.

- As much of the athlete's body as possible should be in the water to allow for the maximum amount of cooling to the entire body (Figure 20-2). This is easier when the water tub is large (ie, 150-gallon Rubbermaid tub). If the tub being used is smaller or if the athlete is larger, rotating ice-water towels to cover the legs and head can maximize cooling.

- While the athlete is being cooled, it is essential to have constant circulation of the water. If the water is not circulated, the temperature of the water next to the skin increases and creates a warm buffer layer that prevents cold water from reaching the skin. Stirring the water continuously introduces cold water to the skin via convection and assists in the rapid cooling of the athlete.

- Once the athlete reaches a core temperature (measured rectally) of 102°F, he or she can be removed from the cold tub and then transported to a nearby hospital for further care.

To maximize the chances of survival in an athlete suffering EHS, it is imperative to aggressively cool the athlete via whole-body CWI. Using the mantra of "cool first, transport second" will allow the clinician to cool the athlete to under 104°F within the first 30 minutes of collapse before further evaluation and treatment in a hospital setting.[2] Every institution sponsoring an athletics program should have CWI incorporated into its policies and procedures manual and emergency action plan. In addition, the sports medicine team should include CWI into their annual training of medical staff, coaches, and emergency medical services personnel to guarantee proper implementation during emergency situations.

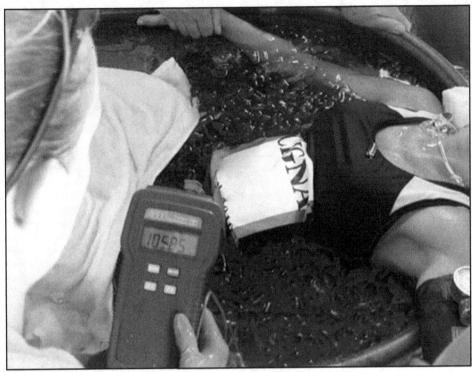

Figure 20-2. EHS victim being cooled during a race.

References

1. Casa DJ, Guskiewicz KM, Anderson SA, et al. National Athletic Trainers' Association position statement: preventing sudden death in sports. *J Athl Train*. 2012;47(1):96-118.
2. Casa DJ, et al. National Athletic Trainers' Association position statement: exertional heat illnesses. *J Athl Train*. 2015;50.
3. Casa DJ, Armstrong LE, Kenny GP, O'Connor FG, Huggins RA. Exertional heat stroke: new concepts regarding cause and care. *Curr Sports Med Rep*. 2012;11(3):115-123.
4. Casa DJ, McDermott BP, Lee EC, Yeargin SW, Armstrong LE, Maresh CM. Cold water immersion: the gold standard for exertional heatstroke treatment. *Exer Sport Sci Rev*. 2007;35(3):141-149.
5. Andersen J, Courson RW, Kleiner DM, McLoda TA. National Athletic Trainers' Association position statement: emergency planning in athletics. *J Athl Train*. 2002;37(1):99-104.

WHAT ARE THE PROPER STEPS FOR THE TREATMENT AND EMERGENCY MANAGEMENT OF AN EXERTIONAL HEAT STROKE VICTIM (INCLUDING APPROPRIATE DURATION OF COOLING AND TRANSPORT TO THE EMERGENCY ROOM)?

Julie K. DeMartini, PhD, ATC and
Robert A. Huggins, PhD, ATC, LAT

Body cooling serves 2 physiological purposes: (1) it returns cooled blood from the skin to the core, which restores cardiovascular function, and (2) it lowers the core body temperature by reducing metabolic rate. The goal for an exertional heat stroke (EHS) victim is to lower the core body temperature to less than 102.5°F (38.9°C) within 30 minutes of collapse.[1] The length of time the core body temperature is above the critical core temperature threshold (105°F/40.5°C) dictates the degree of morbidity and mortality from EHS.[2] Cold-water immersion (CWI) has long been used as the "gold standard" for treatment of EHS and is the most effective cooling modality for patients with EHS.[2-4]

Proper treatment for EHS begins before the incident occurs. Medical staff and coaches should be prepared with the appropriate equipment needed for rapid cooling treatment. On the playing field or in close proximity (such as a nearby locker room or athletic training room), a stock tank, large whirlpool, or kiddie pool should be half filled with water. A sufficient water source should be close by as well as access to ice to keep the water cold. Once an EHS is suspected, prepare to cool the

Lopez RM, ed. *Quick Questions in Heat-Related Illness and Hydration: Expert Advice in Sports Medicine* (pp 111-115).
© 2015 Taylor & Francis Group.

Table 21-1
Checklist for Immediate Care of Exertional Heat Stroke
• Remove athlete from heat and remove equipment/clothing. • Treat if rectal or GI temp is ≥ 104°F or 40.0°C and CNS is altered. • Call 911 and activate emergency action plan. • Immerse victim in ice/cold water tub and aggressively stir water. • If no tub, continuously replace cold wet towels, douse with cold water, and massage ice bags aggressively over entire body. • Cool to 102°F or 38.8°C and monitor vital signs. • Assume a 1°F drop every 3 minutes if no rectal temperature. • After cooling is complete, transport to emergency room.

patient and contact the emergency medical services (EMS). If the tub has not been prepared before the event, fill the tub half way with water, and add ice to make the water temperature between 35°F (1.7°C) and 59°F (15°C). Ice should cover the surface of the water at all times.[3] When assessing a patient with suspected EHS, vital signs including heart rate, blood pressure, respiratory rate, and rectal temperature should be obtained. While assessing the patient's vital signs, central nervous system (CNS) dysfunction should be assessed. Altered CNS symptoms include but are not limited to confusion, dizziness, slurring, and aggression. Once it is confirmed that the patient has a rectal temperature > 104°F (40°C) and that CNS dysfunction is present, excess clothing and athletic equipment should be removed from the body to maximize the skin surface that can be directly cooled. Table 21-1 contains a checklist to prepare the clinician in dealing with a suspected case of EHS.

To begin CWI treatment, the athlete should be placed in the CWI tub. Medical staff, teammates, coaches, and volunteers may be needed to assist with entry of the patient into the tub. Once the patient is in the tub, a towel or sheet may be wrapped across the chest, under the axilla, and pulled together behind the patient's back in an effort to keep the athlete's head from being submerged under the water. (This will be especially helpful if the patient loses consciousness.) Cover as much of the body as possible with the ice water, and if full-body coverage is not possible, the torso should be covered to maximize the surface area being cooled. An ice/wet towel may also be placed over the patient's head and neck while the body is being cooled in the tub. To enhance the temperature gradient between the water and skin (and therefore maximize the cooling potential), the water should be continuously and vigorously stirred.[1,3,4] A large stick or paddle can be used to limit the discomfort of the clinician. If CWI is not available, ice-cold towels should be placed over the entire body surface with repeated cold-water dousing. Another alternative method would be to cover the body completely with ice and continuously pour cold water over top (eg, with a hose or in a locker room shower). During cooling, vital signs and CNS dysfunction should be monitored at regular intervals. Rectal temperature and heart rate should be assessed every 2 minutes, while respiration rate and blood pressure should be assessed every 5 minutes. If a qualified medical professional is available, an intravenous fluid line can be administered for hydration and support of cardiovascular function.

Cooling should continue until the patient's rectal temperature is lowered to 102°F (39°C).[5] This further stresses the importance of acquiring rectal temperature during recognition, as well as continually monitoring throughout treatment.[2] An approximate estimate of cooling when using CWI is 1°C for every 5 minutes and 1°F for every 3 minutes of cooling (assuming the water temperature is less than 60°F and is being aggressively stirred).[1-3] For example, if an athlete has a rectal temperature of 106°F and is placed in a tub for 15 minutes, the body would be expected to cool to approximately 101°F, which is equivalent to a 3°C or 5°F reduction in temperature during that time. However, if we place another athlete at 105°F in the same water and cool for the same duration, that person will be at 100°F and may experience an excessive drop in core temperature. Since individual variability may result in different cooling rates for the same time period, having a rectal temperature device is vital. The rectal temperature will indicate when it is the appropriate time to remove the patient from the tub. However, if rectal temperature cannot be monitored, cool the patient for 10 to 15 minutes and then transport to a medical facility. It is important to note that alternative temperature assessment tools (ie, oral, axillary, tympanic) are not valid indicators of core body temperature in an exercising individual and therefore should not be used. Be aware that even after the cooling treatment has begun, it is not uncommon for the body temperature to remain elevated for the first 3 to 5 minutes. As a matter of fact, it may even continue to increase initially; however, the clinician must continue to stay on course and encourage the sports medicine team to continue cooling the patient aggressively. After the first 5 minutes of cooling, the patient's body temperature will begin to decrease much more rapidly, which is why it is imperative that the athlete remain in the cold tub until the temperature reaches 102°F.

If full-body CWI is not available, partial-body immersion in a small pool/tub and other modalities, such as wet ice towels rotated and placed over the entire body or cold-water dousing with or without fanning, may be used. However, it is important to note that these alternative methods are not as effective as whole-body CWI and may result in suboptimal treatment and a longer cooling time.

If proper cooling via CWI is available, patient transfer to an emergency facility is only indicated after rectal temperature is successfully reduced to 102°F (39°C). This "cool first, transport second" approach is unique to EHS treatment and is critical to ensuring complete and rapid recovery. Emergency medical transport

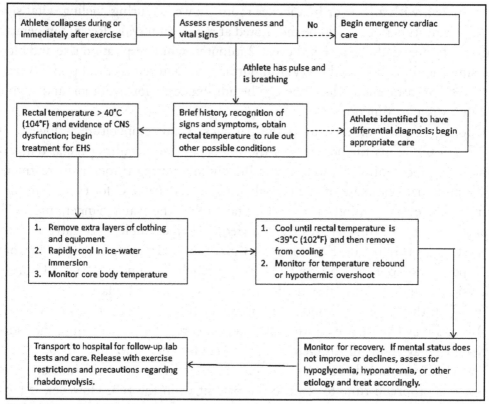

Figure 21-1. Algorithm for treatment of EHS.

services are often trained in emergency conditions to transport patients to the hospital as quickly as possible. With EHS, the time that it takes to transport the patient coupled with the inability to rapidly continue cooling in the ambulance are a recipe for disaster. For example, if CWI is successfully initiated and the EMS team arrives before the athlete has reached 102°F, the clinician must not relinquish care until the treatment is completed. Premature removal may increase the time that a patient is hyperthermic, leading to long-term complications and sequelae. A complete algorithm of EHS treatment can be seen in Figure 21-1. Policies and procedures for cooling athletes before transport to the hospital must be explicitly stated in an emergency action plan and shared with potential EMS responders. This coordinates EHS treatment with all involved medical personnel and limits the possibility of confusion and/or disagreement between parties.

References

1. Casa DJ, Anderson JM, Armstrong LE, Maresh CM. Survival strategy: acute treatment of exertional heat stroke. *J Strength Cond Res.* 2006;20(3):462.
2. Casa DJ, Kenny GP, Taylor NA. Immersion treatment for exertional hyperthermia: cold or temperate water? *Med Sci Sports Exerc.* 2010;42(7):1246-1252.

3. Casa DJ, McDermott BP, Lee EC, et al. Cold water immersion: the gold standard for exertional heatstroke treatment. *Exerc Sport Sci Rev.* 2007;35(3):141-149.
4. Lopez RM, Casa DJ, McDermott BP, Stearns RL, Armstrong LE, Maresh CM. Exertional heat stroke in the athletic setting. *Athl Train Sports Health Care.* 2011;3(4):189-200.
5. Gagnon D, Lemire BB, Casa DJ, Kenny GP. Cold-water immersion and the treatment of hyperthermia: using 38.6°C as a safe rectal temperature cooling limit. *J Athl Train.* 2010;45(5):439-444.

WHAT ARE THE MOST EFFECTIVE ALTERNATIVE METHODS TO COOLING AN EXERTIONAL HEAT STROKE VICTIM IF COLD-WATER IMMERSION IS NOT AVAILABLE?

Julie K. DeMartini, PhD, ATC

The most important determinant in the outcome of exertional heat stroke (EHS) is the amount of time the victim is above the critical threshold for cell damage (40.5°C/105°F). The maximal temperature experienced by the EHS victim is not the most important item, but reducing temperature to less than 40.5°C/105°F in less than 30 minutes is critical for survival.[1] Under a hyperthermic state, effective heat dissipation is facilitated by elevated levels of skin perfusion and sweating; however, whole-body heat loss can be severely compromised in individuals experiencing EHS. Under these conditions, cooling treatments that enhance heat dissipation by increasing conductive heat transfer and/or evaporative heat loss are critical for the survival of the EHS victim.[1]

It is well documented that optimal treatment for EHS is rapid whole-body cold-water immersion (CWI), and treatment should be initiated immediately upon the athlete's collapse.[1-3] However, situations may arise where CWI is not readily available, in which case other methods of body cooling must be considered. Body cooling serves 2 purposes in the treatment of EHS: (1) it lowers core body temperature

Lopez RM, ed. *Quick Questions in Heat-Related Illness and Hydration: Expert Advice in Sports Medicine* (pp 117-121).
© 2015 Taylor & Francis Group.

by reducing the hypermetabolic state of the organs, and (2) it returns blood flow from the skin to the core.[1]

Whole-body cooling methods should be used to reduce body temperature and therefore mitigate damage to the vital organ systems. Cooling rate of the modality used can have a large effect on the amount of time it takes to get the EHS victim under the critical threshold (40.5°C/105°F).[2] Cooling rates for many commonly used modalities are presented in Figure 22-1.[3] Cold-water immersion, the "gold standard" for EHS treatment, is the most effective cooling modality for patients with EHS.[1] The water should be approximately 35°F/1.7°C to 59°F/15°C and continuously stirred to maximize cooling. This method results in the fastest cooling rates reported in the literature[3] and has provided a 100% survival rate when used in various athletic environments.[4] While cooling rates reported in the literature may vary because of differences in study methodology,[3] the cooling rate for CWI when used on EHS victims is approximately 0.37°F/min (0.2°C/min) or about 1°F every 3 minutes (or 1°C every 5 min) when considering the entire immersion period from immediately after collapse until the victim's core body temperature reaches 102°F (39°C).[1,2,4]

If full-body CWI is not available, other cooling modalities must be considered. The cooling modality must not only cool the body rapidly enough to meet the 30-minute criterion, but must also be immediately accessible. In addition to organized athletic teams, another group in which the prevalence of EHS is high is the military, especially during basic training. The military has adopted a modified version of CWI that uses continual ice-water dousing combined with ice massage. This protocol is also commonly practiced at the Marine Corps Marathon, in which a 100% survival rate has also been reported (similar to the 100% survival rate associated with the Falmouth Road Race[4]); however, it is important to note that the cooling rate of this modality is 70% as fast as CWI.[5] For this method, the EHS patient is placed on a porous cot that is suspended over a tub filled with ice water, and the entire body is continuously doused with ice water, while vigorous ice massage of the limbs is simultaneously applied.[5] This method also requires that several personnel are available to provide treatment, as multiple people are necessary to continually douse, massage, and monitor the EHS victim.

A readily portable (and inexpensive) alternative to CWI for scenarios of remote care (or when a tub is not accessible or prepared) is the rotation of ice or wet towels (Figure 22-2). While cooling rates are approximately half of that of CWI (0.10°C/min versus 0.20°C/min, respectively),[3] this method has been shown to be an acceptable alternative for body cooling.[3] For this method to be maximally effective, towels should be kept in a cooler with ice and water until used. With the EHS victim lying supine, individual towels should be placed over the torso, around each arm, around each leg, and over the head. Towels should then be rotated (while the

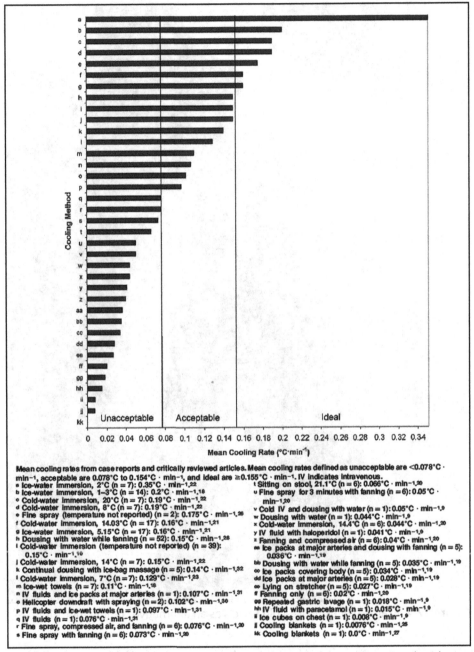

Figure 22-1. Mean cooling rates of various cooling modalities. (Reprinted with permission from McDermott BP, Casa DJ, Ganio MS, et al. Acute whole-body cooling for exercise-induced hyperthermia: a systematic review. *J Athl Train.* 2009;44[1]:84-93.)

victim is also being resubmerged in the ice water) approximately every 2 minutes to provide maximal cooling. This method can also be combined with fanning to maximize the evaporative heat loss potential of the EHS patient.

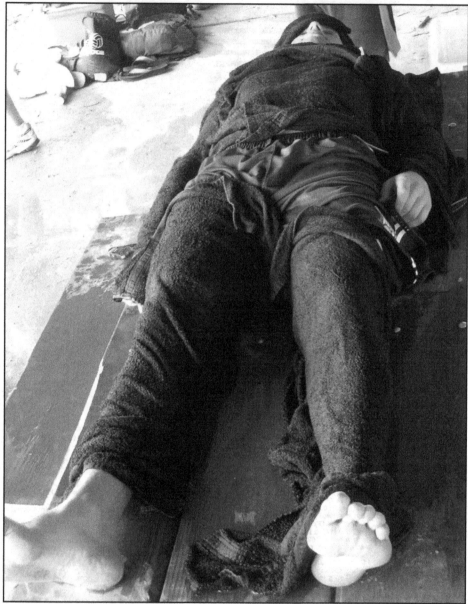

Figure 22-2. Example of using ice-cold towels as an alternative cooling modality.

Two other methods to consider if no other option is available are partial immersion with dousing using a tarp and placing the EHS victim in a cold shower in a locker room. Although cooling rates have not yet been analyzed for these 2 methods, field reports suggest moderate success in reducing core body temperature. The tarp method may be considered if a cooling tub is not available, such as in a remote environment where transporting the tub is not possible and/or there is no available water source (ie, cross-country meet in a remote location). In this case, a tarp can be spread out with its edges suspended, and the EHS victim can be placed on the tarp surrounded by cold/ice water. For the shower method, the EHS victim can be placed in a cold shower with the cold water continuously running over the body. Fanning can accompany this method to promote evaporative heat loss. This method may be used if no cooling modality is available, and the EHS victim is near a locker room or other building in which a shower is available. As part of the appropriate treatment protocol for an EHS victim is "cool first, transport second,"[2] these methods can certainly be considered, especially when more suitable methods are not available.

While other cooling modalities have had variable degrees of success, placing ice bags over peripheral arteries has continually shown to be ineffective and unacceptable for the treatment of EHS.[3] Although this method has been practiced for several years, it is a misconception among many medical professionals that these modalities provide adequate cooling. Therefore, certified athletic trainers and other health care professionals should implement an appropriate emergency action plan to ensure that they are equipped with a more suitable option for the treatment of EHS. While immediate whole-body CWI is the preferred method for treatment of EHS, certified athletic trainers must ensure they have a viable alternative if/when CWI is not available.

References

1. Casa DJ, Armstrong LE, Kenny GP, et al. Exertional heat stroke: new concepts regarding cause and care. *Cur Sports Med Rep.* 2012;11(3):115-123.
2. Pryor RR, Casa DJ, Holschen JC, et al. Exertional heat stroke: strategies for prevention and treatment from the sports field to the emergency department. *Clin Ped Emerg Med.* 2013;14(4):267-278.
3. McDermott BP, Casa DJ, Ganio MS, et al. Acute whole-body cooling for exercise-induced hyperthermia: a systematic review. *J Athl Train.* 2009;44(1):84-93.
4. DeMartini JK, Casa DJ, Belval L, et al. Effectiveness of CWI in the treatment of EHS at the Falmouth Road Race. *Med Sci Sport Exerc.* 2014;June 30. Epub ahead of print.
5. McDermott BP, et al. Cold water dousing with ice massage to treat exertional heat stroke: a case series. *ASEM.* 2009;80(8):720-722.

DOES COLD-WATER IMMERSION CAUSE SHOCK OR OTHER ADVERSE EVENTS?

Lindsey E. Eberman, PhD, LAT, ATC

Although cold-water immersion (CWI) has been well established in the literature as the "gold standard" method of cooling hyperthermic individuals,[1] hesitation and apprehension still exist. Some of the common misconceptions about CWI include effectiveness, discomfort, unsanitary water conditions, lack of feasibility, peripheral vasoconstriction, shivering, hypothermic afterdrop, and difficulty in applying supplemental treatments.[1] Several systematic reviews and position statements have worked to demystify CWI and to eliminate any concerns regarding the potential adverse events among those skeptics.[1,2] The purpose of this response is to further clarify the use of CWI in the treatment of hyperthermic individuals. Treatment of exertional heat stroke (EHS) with rapid, aggressive cooling within 30 minutes of collapse has resulted in an irrefutable survival rate[2]—an unarguable statistic in saving lives from EHS.

Various cooling modalities have been investigated and cited throughout the literature.[2] Although the body of work has not provided a rigorous comparison of modalities with patients experiencing EHS, there is clear evidence that CWI is the

Lopez RM, ed. *Quick Questions in Heat-Related Illness and Hydration: Expert Advice in Sports Medicine* (pp 123-126).
© 2015 Taylor & Francis Group.

gold standard method for rapid cooling of hyperthermic individuals.[2] What may have been formerly acceptable (ie, ice bags over peripheral arteries, fanning, shade, etc) are no longer supported by evidence because of their subpar cooling rates.[1,2] Further, colder water and the use of water circulation have shown the most effective cooling rates for drastically decreasing core body temperature in hyperthermic individuals.[1-3] Some of the other misconceptions can be easily dismissed[1]:

- Discomfort should not be the primary concern of the patient or the practitioner—saving cells from hyperthermic destruction is.

- Unsanitary water conditions can be remedied with solutions that are approved by the Environmental Protection Agency after each use.

- Although the feasibility and availability of an immersion tub "in the field" may be difficult given specific sport, exercise, and occupational situations, those in the athletics community should always be prepared. Alternative cooling modalities may be helpful, as long as they cool at a rate of 0.1°C/min when cooling begins immediately, and no slower than 0.15°C/min if cooling is delayed (> 20 to 30 min).

What seems to remain for those speculating about the negative effects of CWI are peripheral vasoconstriction, shivering, hypothermic afterdrop, and difficulty in applying supplemental treatments (ie, intravenous, automated external defibrillator [AED]). Peripheral vasoconstriction does occur in normothermic individuals, but that is not the case in hyperthermic individuals.[1,2] The best example for exposure to CWI in normothermic individuals is among fisherman working in places like the Bering Sea. In the worst case scenario, they could be exposed to the coldest water in the world and their bodies will respond to protect and maintain core body temperature. Although the protection mechanism is short lived (about 15 to 20 minutes), the periphery will work to protect the core by constricting the vascular structures and shunting blood to the core. This is called the Currie response and refers to both the peripheral vasoconstriction protection mechanisms occurring within the first 8 to 10 minutes of CWI exposure to maintain core temperature stability (Figure 23-1).[1]

In hyperthermic individuals, this same body mechanism does not occur or at least not in a way that prevents cooling,[1] despite popular belief (see Figure 23-1). During a state of hyperthermia, such as with EHS, the hypothalamus is more sensitive to fluctuations in core temperature, not skin temperature. As such, the period of blood being shunted to the core and subsequent rise in core body temperature associated with the Currie effect is negligent (only about 0.1°C to 0.2°C/0.18°F to 0.36°F).[1] It is also not uncommon for the core body temperature of an EHS patient to continue to rise after collapse because of continued metabolic heat production. When utilizing CWI with a hyperthermic athlete, there is a larger temperature

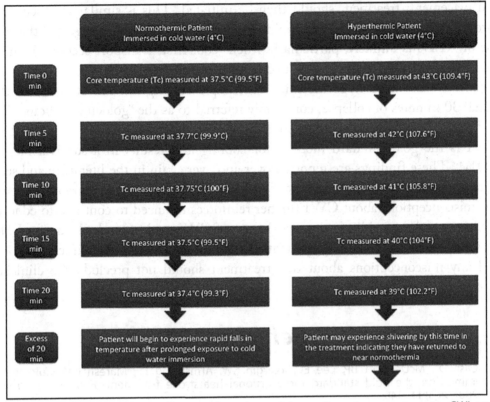

	Normothermic Patient Immersed in cold water (4°C)	Hyperthermic Patient Immersed in cold water (4°C)
Time 0 min	Core temperature (Tc) measured at 37.5°C (99.5°F)	Core temperature (Tc) measured at 43°C (109.4°F)
Time 5 min	Tc measured at 37.7°C (99.9°C)	Tc measured at 42°C (107.6°F)
Time 10 min	Tc measured at 37.75°C (100°F)	Tc measured at 41°C (105.8°F)
Time 15 min	Tc measured at 37.5°C (99.5°F)	Tc measured at 40°C (104°F)
Time 20 min	Tc measured at 37.4°C (99.3°F)	Tc measured at 39°C (102.2°F)
Excess of 20 min	Patient will begin to experience rapid falls in temperature after prolonged exposure to cold water immersion	Patient may experience shivering by this time in the treatment indicating they have returned to near normothermia

Figure 23-1. Comparison of normothermic and hyperthermic responses to CWI at 4°C/39.2°F.

gradient between the ice-cold water temperature and the patient's elevated core temperature, thus allowing for rapid cooling. As core temperature returns to baseline, this gradient decreases and the rate of cooling slows. In practice, 9 minutes of cooling in 2°C/35.6°F CWI can yield cooling to about 38.6°C/101.5°F core body temperature and will prevent overcooling.[4]

In normothermic individuals, shivering is a likely by-product of CWI, simply because we are cooling the skin rapidly.[1] However, in hyperthermic individuals, shivering is not as common,[3] unless they are cooled too long.[1] Hypothermic afterdrop occurs when the EHS victim is excessively cooled. To avoid hypothermic afterdrop, the practitioner should measure core body temperature through a flexible, rectal thermistor until the core temperature has returned to 39°C/102.2°F.[1,5] Continuous monitoring can help prevent hypothermic afterdrop and allow for timely transport following cooling.

The difficulty in applying supplemental treatments is a real one. During immersion it is possible to administer intravenous fluids and supplemental oxygen; however, the use of an AED is far more difficult.[1] In the event an AED is required, the patient should be removed from the tub and dried in the areas necessary for pad placement; treatment should then be initiated. This is similar to rescuing a cardiac arrest victim from a swimming pool. The literature has suggested that the use of AEDs is unlikely, particularly when "cool first, transport second" is initiated early.[1] AEDs are likely only necessary when end-organ damage is occurring because of prolonged hyperthermia, when rapid cooling has not occurred in the initial 30 minutes of collapse, commonly referred to as the "golden half-hour."[1,2]

The use of an effective cooling modality in the treatment of EHS is essential.[1,2,5] CWI is the gold standard method for cooling and results in a survival rate of 100%.[1-5] These findings are reported over and over again in the literature and seen in real-life cases of EHS. The lack of literature or case studies to support the various misconceptions about CWI further reinforces the need to continue to educate clinicians and the public to support the use of CWI as the standard care for EHS patients.[1-4] CWI to treat EHS patients is the best evidence-based clinical practice, and any misconceptions about this treatment should not preclude the clinician from delivering the best care.

References

1. Casa DJ, McDermott BP, Lee EC, Yeargin SW, Armstrong LE, Maresh CM. Cold water immersion: the gold standard for exertional heatstroke treatment. *Exerc Sport Sci Rev.* 2007;35(3):141-149.
2. McDermott BP, Casa DJ, Ganio MS, et al. *J Athl Train.* 2009;44(1):84-93.
3. Proulx CI, Ducharme MB, Kenny GP. Effect of water temperature on cooling efficiency during hyperthermia in humans. *J Appl Physiol.* 2003;94(4):1317-1323.
4. Gagnon D, Lemire BB, Casa DJ, Kenny GP. Cold-water immersion and the treatment of hyperthermia: using 38.6°C as a safe rectal temperature cooling limit. *J Athl Train.* 2010;45(5):439-444.
5. Casa DJ, et al. National Athletic Trainers' Association position statement: exertional heat illnesses. *J Athl Train.* 2015;50.

SECTION IV

SPECIAL CONSIDERATIONS
ENVIRONMENTAL CONDITIONS AND RETURN TO PLAY

CAN EXERTIONAL HEAT ILLNESSES OCCUR IN COOL OR COLD ENVIRONMENTS?

Rebecca L. Stearns, PhD, ATC

While more common in hot weather conditions, many factors can contribute to an exertional heat illness. One factor is the intensity of an athlete's exercise session, which can raise an athlete's body temperature faster and higher than potentially any other factor. This helps explain how exertional heat illnesses, more commonly exertional heat stroke (EHS), still occurs in cooler weather conditions. This section will address these possibilities within the spectrum of potential heat illnesses.

An early study by Saltin and Hermansen[1] demonstrated the large difference in body temperature response to a range of intensities in temperate weather conditions (19°C to 22°C/66°F to 72°F).[1] In this study, body temperature increased about 0.5°C/0.9°F for every additional 25% increase in intensity (based on VO_2max).[1] Thereby, if a subject started at normal body temperature (37°C/98.6°F), working at 25% of his or her maximum exercise capacity would increase body temperature to 37.5°C, 50% would increase body temperature to 38°C, and 75% to 38.5°C (101.3°F). This study clearly demonstrated the impact of exercise intensity on body temperature responses. While this same experiment has not been reproduced in cold environments, it is likely that this response is similar, though probably to a lesser degree.

Lopez RM, ed. *Quick Questions in Heat-Related Illness and Hydration: Expert Advice in Sports Medicine* (pp 129-132).

Race Description	Starting Race Temperature	Reported Cases of Heat Stroke	Reference
Table 24-1 **Various Races and Starting Race Temperatures for Cool Weather Exertional Heat Stroke Cases**			
10-mile race	5°C/41°F	3	4
Half marathon (13.1 miles)	14°C/57°F	3	4
Marathon (26.2 miles)	6°C/43°F	1	3

Complementing this study was another by Mora-Rodriguez et al,[2] who examined the impact of variable-intensity exercise versus constant exercise intensity on body temperature response. In this study, alternating between 90% and 50% of VO_2max produced greater heat storage, rectal temperatures, and heart rates compared with an equal workload completed at 60% of VO_2max.[2] This demonstrates that incorporation of intense exercise, even with intermittent bouts of lower-intensity exercise, creates a higher thermal stress than a constant lower-intensity exercise.

While few examples exist, there are case reports of athletes exercising at high exercise intensity (mainly road races) resulting in severe hyperthermia and cases of EHS, even in the midst of cool weather. One case report outlined a marathon runner in his 30s collapsing just before the finish line.[3] Though the race started at 8 am when it was 6°C/43°F, the runner succumbed to EHS with an initial (although delayed approximately 27 min) rectal temperature of 40.7°C/105.3°F.[3] In another report of 2 races with cool-weather heat stroke cases, 3 runners collapsed at a half marathon, with a starting race temperature of 14°C/57°F, while 3 other runners succumbed to heat stroke in a 10-mile race where air temperature remained between 5°C and 9°C/41°F and 48°F.[4] Table 24-1 summarizes these cases and the factors present for each. It should also be noted that for many spring or fall races, the predicted starting race temperatures can change quickly. The potential for a participant to overdress for the weather is a very possible scenario, in which case the extra clothing could increase the heat load, even in cooler weather conditions.

While it is clear that high-intensity exercise can quickly increase body temperature up to the point of EHS, even in cool weather, there is very little to no literature in regard to other heat illnesses (ie, heat exhaustion, heat syncope, and heat cramps). Heat exhaustion and heat syncope are both conditions that result from an imbalance of blood distribution because of a high blood demand from the skin and working muscles. Maintaining appropriate blood volume will be largely dependent on the appropriate intake of water and electrolytes. Consequently, water and electrolyte loss via sweat presents a major threat to blood volume maintenance during exercise.[5] Normal sweat losses for athletes can range from 0.5 to 2.0 L/hour (depending on the athlete's size, sex, fitness, and environmental conditions).[5] This explains why it is very easy during a longer event for athletes to lose fluids and electrolytes, reducing blood volume at a time of greatest demand. Therefore, the scenario that most likely places an athlete at risk for a heat exhaustion or heat syncope event in cool weather is one where an individual is exercising very intensely for a prolonged period, he or she overdresses for the weather conditions, becomes dehydrated, and loses a large amount of sodium, all of which would result in a decrease in blood volume. While the cause for heat cramps is a debated topic, the proposed factors that could result in heat cramps (ie, intense exercise, dehydration, sweat and sodium losses) are also present in cold weather and are therefore possible outcomes from athletic participation.

Overall, while heat illness is much less likely to occur in conditions of cool weather, it is possible for it to occur. It is important to consider all factors when assessing a collapsed athlete in any weather. In cooler environments, more elite athletes who are able to participate at high exercise intensities for long-distance events are possibly more at risk for heat illness (particularly EHS) compared with slower athletes who may finish later and be more susceptible to a cold injury. In such a case it is very possible to have the need to treat both hyperthermic and hypothermic athletes in the medical tent for the same event. This also highlights the need for accurate assessment devices. It has been anecdotally reported that in some cases of heat stroke that occurred in cool-weather marathons, an inaccurate temperature measurement device was used, leading the diagnoses to hypothermia as opposed to hyperthermia, ultimately delaying critical care. This is why it is critical for medical providers to understand the dynamics of heat production and heat loss in athletes and keep an open mind in order to consider all contributing factors when an athlete arrives for medical care, even in a cool environment.

References

1. Saltin B, Hermansen L. Esophageal, rectal and muscle temperature during exercise. *J Appl Physiol*. 1966;21(6):1757-1762.
2. Mora-Rodriguez R, Del Coso J, Estevez E. Thermoregulatory responses to constant versus variable-intensity exercise in the heat. *Med Sci Sports Exerc*. 2008;40(11):1945-1952.
3. Roberts WO. Exertional heat stroke during a cool weather marathon: a case study. *Med Sci Sports Exerc*. 2006;38(7):1197-1203.

4. Robertson B, Walter E. "Cool runnings": heat stroke in cool conditions. *Emerg Med J.* 2010;27:387-388.
5. American College of Sports Medicine, Sawka MN, Burke LM, et al. American College of Sports Medicine position stand: exercise and fluid replacement. *Med Sci Sports Exerc.* 2007;39(2):377-390.

WHAT ARE THE BEST METHODS OF ASSESSING ENVIRONMENTAL CONDITIONS AND WHAT MODIFICATIONS SHOULD BE MADE TO WORK-TO-REST RATIOS, PRACTICES, AND GAMES BASED ON THE ENVIRONMENT?

Earl R. "Bud" Cooper, EdD, ATC, CSCS

Environmental stress has been a focus of attention over the past few years as cases of heat-related deaths have been on the rise. Grundstein et al[1] reviewed mortality rates among football participants that were hyperthermic in nature. Over the past 30 years (1980 to 2009), these mortality rates have almost tripled. The majority of these deaths occurred in the fall months, when the atmospheric conditions tended to be warmer; 71% of the August deaths occurred in the first 2 weeks of the month, which typically correlate with the first 2 weeks of football practice when the student athletes are beginning to acclimatize to the environment.

Exertional heat illness (EHI) is a fairly common occurrence in sporting events, particularly in the fall season. Numerous investigators have advocated preventative measures to lessen the risk of EHI; however, it is difficult to pinpoint the best solution when there is no direct cause-and-effect relationship when modifying a single variable such as hot temperatures. If we are to target one of the variables to modify, altering practice start times to when weather conditions are less stressful may be a good place to begin. Currently, environmental conditions have been measured by one of 2 methods: heat index (HI) and wet bulb globe temperature (WBGT). While the

Lopez RM, ed. *Quick Questions in Heat-Related Illness and Hydration: Expert Advice in Sports Medicine* (pp 133-136).

HI is probably the most well known, it is the least applicable to the sports population. The HI assessment (ambient air temperature and humidity) is the National Weather Service's assessment of the apparent temperature and has been in use for more than 3 decades. The HI is based on environmental measurements taken in the shade with a person of standard stature (5'7", 147 lb) wearing long pants and a short sleeve shirt, and walking at a rate of 3 mph. While this method of environmental stress measurement is appropriate for the general population, this description is not applicable to the sporting population. Additionally, the HI does not include the assessment of radiant heat, which is a significant variable when determining heat stress. Currently, HI has not been endorsed by any of the major sports medicine associations for use with specific athletic populations. While HI scales have been used by state high school athletic associations, to date none of these scales are "national norms" and do not base their recommendations on data-driven research. Additionally, they do not include recommendations to specific age group populations.

The WBGT, on the other hand, is widely accepted by many prestigious organizations (American College of Sports Medicine [ACSM], American Academy of Pediatrics, Department of Defense [DOD]) as a more accurate measurement of environmental stress. The WBGT takes into account ambient air temperature and humidity as well as radiant heating effects (important when considering playing surfaces such as artificial grass and "SuperTurf"). Each of these variables is weighted differently. The calculation is based on the following formula: $WBGT = 0.7T_{wb} + 0.2T_{bg} + 0.1 T_{db}$. Wet bulb (humidity) is the most influential (because of its negative effect on the body's ability to cool via the sweating mechanism), followed by black globe (radiant heat) and then dry temperature (ambient air temperature).[2] The ACSM[3] and DOD have both developed a WBGT index that recommends variations of activity and work-rest ratios according to the environment's level of heat stress. Due to varying climates in different regions of the country, regional WBGT readings should be used as the guiding variable when making decisions on the number of rest breaks and the activity intensity and duration.[2] Essentially, as the level of heat increases, the risk of EHI rises, especially for those who have been identified as positive for sickle cell trait or are nonacclimatized; therefore, precautionary steps should be taken.

The WBGT can be measured with a WBGT monitor. This device ranges in price from as low as $200 to $4500. Reliability and accuracy of these units will depend largely on following the manufacturer's instructions (turning the unit on approximately 15 minutes prior to use to allow it to adjust to current weather conditions, taking WBGT readings in a sunny area near where activity will take place, and making periodic measurements during activity). It is recommended that WBGT measurements be taken at least 3 times during an activity session (beginning, middle, and near the end) to ensure that the environmental stress has not increased and placed a more significant load on the athlete. While utilization of the WBGT index has been

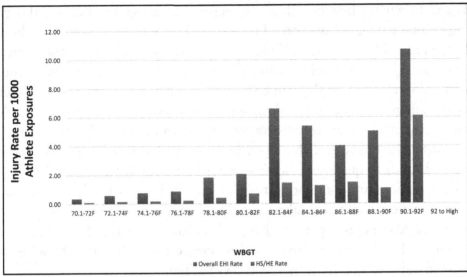

Figure 25-1. EHI rate based on WBGT Index readings.

recognized as the "gold standard" when it comes to environmental assessments, how does it compare with other instruments used by clinicians in the field? The HI, as mentioned previously, has been shown to have its limitations by sheer definition and application guidelines. The sling psychrometer is another device often used in the field that measures humidity and ambient air temperature similar to the HI. Both of these measures neglect the importance of assessing the radiant heat (black globe)—the second most influential measurement of WBGT.

Developing appropriate work-to-rest ratios for participating athletes is critical to preventing the onset of any type of EHI, such as heat exhaustion or heat stroke. Part of any prevention strategy is ensuring that the athletes are properly acclimatized to the atmospheric conditions. This includes a gradual exposure to the environmental conditions as well as strict limits on the length of activity and amount of equipment worn during times of environmental stress. The National Collegiate Athletic Association,[4] National Athletic Trainers' Association (NATA),[2] and ACSM offer specific guidelines for football practices beginning each fall. In addition, numerous high school associations have implemented specific policies regarding these practices. Establishing proper work-rest ratios and fluid replacement volumes will sustain performance and help to stave off EHIs. Avoiding the hottest part of the day for practice sessions is another key component to reduce these risks. Midday (12 to 4 pm) is traditionally the hottest part of the day and should be avoided if at all possible; providing access to hydration stations throughout practices will also help to lower risk. Previous research[5] has indicated that EHI risk will increase as the WBGT rises, thereby advocating practice times be held during a cooler part of the day (Figure 25-1). Allowing players to remove equipment during conditioning drills and to remove helmets when not engaged in active practice are also good strategies, as is having a "cool zone" for those athletes who may succumb to heat. A cool zone can easily be set up by designating an area of shade where the distressed athlete is out of direct sunlight. Items to have on hand in this area include containers with cold water and ice that can be used to cool down the athlete using sponges or towels wrung out over the athlete, large fans to assist with evaporative cooling, water/misting stations, or ice tubs for total body immersion. The NATA recommends that an ice tub be available *on site* in the event that an athlete lapses into heat stroke and needs to quickly reduce his or her core body temperature. Identifying at-risk populations and monitoring them closely during practice/games is another important tactic to employ. Athletes should always be given formal rest/hydration breaks every 20 minutes of practice, have a shady location to rest during breaks, and be encouraged to drink a minimum of 4 to 6 ounces of fluids. Rest breaks should increase in duration and frequency as the WBGT increases.

Having the ability to accurately measure environmental conditions, knowing your athletic population (at-risk individuals, acclimatization status, and pre-existing conditions), and having a proper practice policy for hot environments will help lessen the risk of heat illnesses and potential catastrophic events.

References

1. Grundstein AJ, Ramseyer C, Zhao F, et al. A retrospective analysis of American football hyperthermia deaths in the United States. *Int J Biometeorol*. 2010;Dec. Epub.
2. Casa DJ, et al. National Athletic Trainers' Association position statement: exertional heat illnesses. *J Athl Train*. 2015;50.
3. American College of Sports Medicine. American College of Sports Medicine position stand on exertional heat illness during training and competition. *Med Sci Sports Exerc*. 2007;556-572.
4. National Collegiate Athletic Association. *NCAA Heat Acclimation Policy: 2003-04 NCAA Division I manual*. Indianapolis, IN: Author; 2003.
5. Cooper ER, Broglio SP, Casa DJ, Miles JD, Powell JW, Ferrara MS. Risk rates of exertional heat illness among intercollegiate football players. *J Athl Train*. In review.

QUESTION 26

WHEN CAN AN ATHLETE RETURN TO PLAY FOLLOWING AN EXERTIONAL HEAT ILLNESS?

Robert A. Huggins, PhD, ATC, LAT and
Francis G. O'Connor, MD, MPH

Return to play (RTP) is defined as the progression back to full activity following an illness or injury. The main goals of RTP are safety and timeliness. Therefore, this complex decision must be made only after proper evaluation, treatment, and rehabilitation have been performed under proper supervision. The American College of Sports Medicine has recommended guidelines on RTP[1,2] with the primary goal of safe return to activity in mind. The following criteria must be considered to promote proper and effective return to activity:

- Status of anatomic function and healing
- Status of recovery from the illness and long-term effects
- Status of the ongoing injury or illness
- Level of risk posed to other participants
- Return of sport-specific skills
- Psychosocial readiness

Lopez RM, ed. *Quick Questions in Heat-Related Illness and
Hydration: Expert Advice in Sports Medicine* (pp 137-142).
© 2015 Taylor & Francis Group.

- Ability to perform with equipment and/or braces
- Compliance with federal, state, local, school, and sport governing bodies

The RTP of athletes suffering from an exertional heat illness needs to be made by a health care professional trained in the prevention, diagnosis, and treatment of heat illnesses. Athletic trainers, medical doctors, and doctors of osteopathic medicine are qualified in heat illness care and management and should be consulted before making an RTP decision. Effectively making an RTP decision following heat illness requires an understanding of the pathophysiology of the body as well as the recovery of the body systems. This chapter will overview common types of heat illness as well as the RTP criteria for each.

Heat Cramps

Heat cramps are spasms or twitches of the muscle that result from large sodium and water loss during exercise in the heat.[3] Often heat cramps appear as muscle spasms and subside within minutes if fluid and sodium are replaced.

RTP following heat cramps often can occur as soon as the cramp resolves or following the replacement of fluids and rest. Players can return to the game or match in the same day. When cramping is prolonged, it may take up to 24 hours to RTP. If the player reports the next day with muscle soreness, the intensity and volume of exercise should be modified to minimize further muscle damage. If cramping or pain continues >24 hours, serologic and urine markers of muscle damage such as blood urea nitrogen, creatinine, and myoglobin should be considered. Furthermore, diet analysis (specifically sodium intake) should be examined to identify any possible deficit, and sodium supplementation may be warranted.

Heat Syncope

Syncope is commonly defined as a fainting episode. There are many types of syncope, with their clinical presentation being the determining factor for classification. Heat syncope is often the result of hypotension that results from pooling of the blood in the extremities and often occurs from standing in an upright posture or inadequate heat acclimatization. Heat syncope will often occur during the first few days of heat exposure, before adaptations of the cardiovascular system have taken place. During the first 1 to 3 days of heat exposure, increased blood to the skin occurs, causing blood pooling in the extremities. Deceases in blood pressure and decreased oxygen levels to the brain result in fainting.

RTP following heat syncope can often occur within the same exercise session as long as the patient is mentating normally and body temperature is not dangerously elevated (> 104°F). The underlying problem (often cardiovascular insufficiency) will take 4 to 7 days of heat acclimatization. While the condition is acute, it is recommended that athletes stay hydrated and avoid standing still immediately following intense exercise. At rest if blood sugar (normally 70 to 100 mg/dL), blood pressure (normally 120/80 mm Hg), pulse (normally approximately 60 to 100 bpm), or respiration rate (normally 8 to 16 breaths/min) are outside of their normal range, the athlete should be withheld from activity. If all vital signs are within normal ranges, the athlete may be permitted to RTP. If repeated episodes of heat syncope occur, a medical provider should examine the athlete to ensure there are no underlying cardiac issues, hypoglycemia, or medication-derived mechanisms causing collapse. Any syncopal or presyncopal event associated with exertion should be cleared by the team physician before RTP is permitted.

Heat Exhaustion

Dehydration and increased body mass index are commonly associated with heat exhaustion. Heat exhaustion is the inability to continue exercise in the heat and is the most common heat-related illness.[1] Heat exhaustion is often an issue of inadequate blood volume. RTP following heat exhaustion should not be permitted within 24 hours. The athlete should have adequate rest, and hydration status should be returned to normal pre-exercising levels based on the following:

- Urine color is a light yellow or straw color
- Body mass is within 1% to 2% of patient's normal pre-exercising values
- Urine specific gravity denotes euhydration, < 1.020
- Plasma osmolality within 285 to 300 mOsm/kg

Furthermore, proper education of the athlete's nutritional and dietary habits should be considered. Increases in dietary sodium and daily fluid intake, as well as replacing adequate water losses during and after exercise, should be emphasized.

Most athletes can RTP after approximately 24 to 48 hours; however, athletes with complications (ie, persistent headache, fatigue at rest or upon initial return to exercise) should refrain from activity until signs and symptoms of dehydration cease.

Sweat rate and electrolyte testing should be considered with recurrent heat exhaustion episodes to quantify the athlete's losses and provide accurate recommendations for fluid and electrolyte supplementation. In recurrent cases, heat tolerance testing may be warranted to determine if the athlete is capable of proper thermoregulation (indicated by a plateau of heart rate and core body temperature) during exercise.

Table 26-1

Normal Laboratory Blood Measures for Return to Play From Exertional Heat Stroke

Blood or Serum Enzyme Measure	BUN (mg/dL)	Creatinine (mg/dL)	AST (UI/L)	ALT (UI/L)	CK (UI/L)	LDH (UI/L)
Normal level*	5 to 20	0.6 to 1.2; M 0.5 to 1.1; F	<40	<31; F BMI ≤ 23[†] <42; F BMI ≥ 23[†] <41; M BMI ≤ 23[†] <66; M BMI ≥ 23[†]	45 to 260	<250

* Specific ranges should be established for each laboratory to determine abnormal ranges for each of the markers above.

† Values adjusted to BMI and sex.

Abbreviations: ALT, alanine transaminase; AST, aspartate aminotransferase; BMI, body mass index; BUN, blood urea nitrogen; CK, creatine kinase; F, female; g/dL, grams per deciliter; LDH, lactate dehydrogenase; M, male; UI/L, international units per liter.

Exertional Heat Stroke

Exertional heat stroke (EHS) is a medical emergency and occurs when 2 criteria are met: body temperature is increased to ≥40.5°C or 105°F and central nervous system dysfunction is present. Current RTP guidelines in sport and the military[4,5] are based on the return of the athlete to normal mentation and a restoration of normal end-organ function (eg, liver [liver function tests], kidney [blood urea nitrogen and creatinine], muscle [creatine kinase]). As normal laboratory blood measures can vary based upon gender, race, baseline activity level, time of day, and individual laboratories, clinical judgment must be used in assessing a return to normal. Once these parameters have been determined to be normal, an athlete may begin a graduated RTP with careful attention to acclimatization. These RTP recommendations, however, are supported by limited research and most are based on common-sense guidelines.[4] Commonly reported values for blood and serum enzyme measures are included in Table 26-1. Normal range for any laboratory test is the mean value of healthy individuals ± 2 SD or the mean ± 95%. These values should be interpreted in the context of the individual athlete.

Table 26-2		
Criteria for Return to Play Following Exertional Heat Illness		
Type of Exertional Heat Illness	**Primary Criteria**	**Secondary Criteria**
Heat cramps	Resolution of cramping	Normal urinary measures if symptoms > 24 hours
Heat syncope	Normal mentation and core body temperature < 104°F	Normal vital signs (eg, BP, pulse, RR)
Heat exhaustion	Return to normal hydration status using %BML, USG, urine color, or plasma osmolality	Consider modification of fluid intake and dietary sodium supplementation
Heat stroke	Demonstrates no sequelae	Normal blood and liver enzymes
Abbreviations: %BML, percent body mass loss; BP, blood pressure; RR, respiration rate; RTP, return to play; USG, urine specific gravity.		

Many of the current guidelines are not evidence based. RTP following EHS can range anywhere from 1 week to 15 months. This widely reported range has led medical professionals and researchers to develop individualized plans for their athletes similar to concussion RTP. The RTP following EHS involves detailed planning with gradually increasing stress on the body. The process should be developed and implemented by an athletic trainer and/or physician.

Conclusion

Research in the area of RTP following exertional heat illnesses is lacking, and current recommendations are largely based on the intuition of the clinician, on a patient-by-patient basis. When an emergency condition (eg, EHS) is ruled out, athletes with conditions such as heat syncope, heat cramps, and heat exhaustion often can RTP with proper hydration and normal vital signs. When episodes recur, patients should be referred for further evaluation and clearance by a physician. Following EHS, a more conservative RTP progression with close monitoring is warranted and should be overseen by a health care professional and/or health care team (eg, MD, DO, AT, LPRN). Serological laboratory blood measures and heat tolerance testing are recommended when considering return to strenuous physical activity (Table 26-2).

References

1. Armstrong LE, Casa DJ, Millard-Stafford M, Moran DS, Pyne SW, Roberts WO. American College of Sports Medicine position stand: exertional heat illness during training and competition. *Med Sci Sports Exerc.* 2007;39(3):556-572. doi:10.1249/MSS.0b013e31802fa199.
2. Armstrong LE. *Exertional Heat Illnesses.* Champaign, IL: Human Kinetics; 2003.
3. Bergeron MF. Heat cramps: fluid and electrolyte challenges during tennis in the heat. *J Sci Med Sport Sports Med Aust.* 2003;6(1):19-27.
4. McDermott BP, Casa DJ, Yeargin SW, Ganio MS, Armstrong LE, Maresh CM. Recovery and return to activity following exertional heat stroke: considerations for the sports medicine staff. *J Sport Rehabil.* 2007;16(3):163-181.
5. O'Connor FG, Williams AD, Blivin S, Heled Y, Deuster P, Flinn SD. Guidelines for return to duty (play) after heat illness: a military perspective. *J Sport Rehabil.* 2007;16(3):227-237.

What Is the Proper Functional Progression for an Athlete Returning to Play Following Exertional Heat Stroke?

Brendon P. McDermott, PhD, ATC

Recognition and treatment of exertional heat stroke (EHS) have improved in recent years. Evidence-based recommendations on how to guide patients back into full activity following EHS are limited, so making decisions is tough for clinicians.[1,2]

Following EHS, patients should be evaluated and cleared by appropriately trained physicians to assure no lasting sequelae.[1-3] Following this evaluation, a gradual onset of activity and heat stress should be followed.[1,3,4] Heat stress is quantified by 3 potential factors. One is the environment, another is the amount of metabolic heat being produced by the athlete, and the last is the use of protective equipment that may impede thermoregulation. Ambient temperature and humidity independently contribute to thermal strain and together can create insurmountable heat stress. The more intense the work that is completed during exercise, or the longer the duration of activity, the more metabolic heat is produced by the body. Becoming accustomed to exercise and the heat (heat acclimatization) is one of the most impressive adaptations of human physiology. Further, this represents the best protection against EHS recurrence.[3]

Lopez RM, ed. *Quick Questions in Heat-Related Illness and Hydration: Expert Advice in Sports Medicine* (pp 143-147).

Table 27-1	
Symptoms of Heat Illness	
• Overwhelming fatigue	• Intestinal cramps
• Overwhelming heat	• Weakness
• Nausea/vomiting	• Drowsiness
• Headache	• Irritability
• Dizziness/lightheadedness	• Confusion
• Chills	• Diarrhea
• Anorexia	• Apathy
If any of these symptoms are reported during or as a result of exercise heat stress, the patient should return to the last successful day without symptoms prior to progressing further.	

During exercise progression, it is recommended that patients be monitored closely. Patients should be questioned regarding heat symptoms daily (Table 27-1). If patients experience symptoms during or following activity, the functional progression must allow for complete recovery prior to further progression. Subjective measures such as fatigue, muscle pain, and perceived exertion can aid the process of grading exercise intensity.

Beyond clinical symptoms, the medical professional overseeing functional progression should consider monitoring physiological measures during the patient's return to activity. Body temperature and heart rate can be easily monitored during functional progression. A variety of heart rate monitors are widely available and provide reliable and valid measures. Body temperature can be monitored via an ingestible thermistor. To use these devices, a pill must be ingested 5 to 6 hours prior to activity to assure that the thermistor has entered the intestines. This allows monitoring without artifact from cold fluid ingestion during activity. These measures, taken every 15 to 30 minutes throughout activity, provide data for the clinician overseeing functional progression. Over time, for a given heat stress and exercise intensity, heart rate and body temperature should be lower, demonstrating heat and exercise acclimatization. Further, a safety cutoff of 90% maximal heart rate or core temperature of 39.5°C should prompt the decision to end an athlete's session.

The following represents a suggested functional progression for return to activity for patients following EHS. The progression should occur after physician clearance and under the supervision of an athletic trainer. It is important to note that this progression is based on consistent environmental stress (heat and humidity). This protocol can be used given consistent weather conditions and exposure, but caution should be taken if environmental extremes are present during or following the progression. Further, it is important for the athletic trainer overseeing this progression

Return to Activity Following EHS Data Sheet

Patient's Name: _____   EHS Date: _____

Day of Protocol: _____   Date: _____

WBGT:

90% max HR:

Exercise protocol:

	Pre-ex	15'	30'	45'	60'	75'	90'	105'	120'	135'	150'	165'	180'
HR													
Temp													
RPE													

Muscle pain:

Fatigue:

Signs/symptoms during or following exercise:

Comments/notes:

Figure 27-1. Sample data sheet for functional return to activity following EHS.

to document specifics regarding exercises and available physiological measures (Figure 27-1). This progression should not include timed or highly motivated activity with consequences if performance expectations are not met.

Day 1: Light activity (50% to 60%; eg, using a stationary bike or jogging) should be performed for no more than 30 minutes, and no protective equipment should be used.[4] It is important to consider that, most often, folks having recovered from EHS are not heat-acclimatized like their teammates when they initially return to activity. This is due to the recommended 7-day rest period and follow-up blood work used to clear patients for activity.[4] This activity is not meant to stress them much at all.

Days 2 to 4: The patient should be assessed based on responses from Day 1 of the functional progression. If the patient was not overly fatigued and responded accordingly during and after activity on Day 1, the patient should progress to Day 2. These days should include moderate activity (50% to 60%) for up to 1 hour with no protective equipment. An example would be a 5- to 10-minute warm-up, 5 minutes of jogging, 10 minutes of sport-specific drills at one-half to three-quarter speed, sit-ups, push-ups, 5-minute rest, 10 minutes of sport-specific drills at half speed, and a 10-minute cool-down. These activities are meant to stress the body and thermoregulatory system at a minimal level. A quick assessment to document sweat rate should be completed on Day 2. This will be used to document heat acclimatization later.

Days 5 to 7: These days should include moderate (50% to 75%) activity for up to 1.5 hours without protective equipment. By this time, the initial responses of heat acclimatization are present (plasma volume expansion, sweat rate increases, etc). The activity here should include a thorough warm-up, cool-down, and adequate rest breaks. Sport-specific drills are acceptable provided they are completed at recommended speeds and effort. This will limit heat production and allow time for the thermoregulatory system to acclimatize.

Days 8 to 10: Day 8 is the first day when protective equipment is introduced. Patients who do not require protective equipment should skip Days 8 to 10 in the progression and go from Day 7 to Day 11. Activity should be light to moderate (40% to 65%) with half of the protective equipment (helmet and shoulder pads for football) used for up to 1.5 hours.

Day 11: Activity duration remains the same but should progress in intensity to moderate to intense (70% to 90%) using half the protective equipment for up to 1.5 hours.

Day 12: This day should replicate Day 2 for activity, include no pads, and include an assessment of sweat rate repeated. This should demonstrate an increased sweating rate with the same activity and heat stress.

Day 13: Full protective equipment should be used with moderate activity (60% to 80%) for up to 2 hours. Activity here is almost full speed, and thermal stress is moderate. Adequate warm-up, cool-down, and rest breaks are essential. Sport-specific anaerobic and/or aerobic activity up to 80% effort is recommended.

Day 14: The final day of progression/clearance should involve intense activity (80% to 100%) for the full duration of practice (no more than 3 h). Essentially, this is a full-activity day with monitoring. This day should confirm suspicions of full recovery for the patient. The patient should be able to perform activities on Day 14 with normal body temperature, heart rate, fatigue, heat symptoms, etc, with heat exposure and equipment according to sport specificity.

If, on any of the progression days listed previously, or on the following day, symptoms reappear (see Table 27-1) or a safety cut point is reached, a full evaluation is recommended. Again, medical conditions, medications, diet, hydration, sleep patterns, psychological stress, etc, should be questioned. If there is no likely cause of delayed recovery, and the patient recovers with 1 day of rest, the last day completed without symptoms should be repeated, and the progression continued from that point. If there is recurrence of symptoms 2 or more times in the progression, repeated physician evaluation and perhaps heat-tolerance testing are warranted.[1]

The previous functional progression takes into consideration a gradual onset of protective equipment, exercise intensity, and duration, as well as heat stress. There is some evidence of transient compromised heat tolerance following EHS. However, in most cases, a myriad of causes combine at the onset of EHS, and heat intolerance is not common (~2%).[3,5]

Conclusion

Following appropriate medical clearance, the athletic trainer must use caution in overseeing return to activity for the EHS patient. The suggested functional progression represents the latest in evidence but lacks support from large populations. However, if this progression is followed, documented, and well supervised, the patient should be able to safely return to activity in the heat following EHS. The progression presented here allows the clinician to facilitate positive physiological responses, and the patient will be better protected against future EHS.

References

1. McDermott BP, Casa DJ, Yeargin SW, Ganio MS, Armstrong LE, Maresh CM. Recovery and return to activity following exertional heat stroke: considerations for the sports medicine staff. *J Sport Rehabil.* 2007;16(3):163-181.
2. O'Connor FG, Casa DJ, Bergeron MF, et al. American College of Sports Medicine roundtable on exertional heat stroke—return to duty/return to play: conference proceedings. *Curr Sports Med Rep.* 2010;9(5):314-321.
3. Johnson EC, Kolkhorst FW, Richburg A, Schmitz A, Martinez J, Armstrong LE. Specific exercise heat stress protocol for a triathlete's return from exertional heat stroke. *Curr Sports Med Rep.* 2013;12(2):106-109.
4. Armstrong LE, Casa DJ, Millard-Stafford M, Moran DS, Pyne SW, Roberts WO. American College of Sports Medicine position stand: exertional heat illness during training and competition. *Med Sci Sports Exerc.* 2007;39(3):556-572.
5. Rav-Acha M, Hadad E, Epstein Y, Heled Y, Moran DS. Fatal exertional heat stroke: a case series. *Am J Med Sci.* 2004;328(2):84-87.

SECTION V

HYDRATION

WHAT ARE THE MOST PRACTICAL, VALID METHODS OF MEASURING HYDRATION STATUS IN ATHLETES?

Michelle A. Cleary, PhD, ATC

A variety of clinical/field techniques exist for athletic trainers to determine hydration status. Optimal physical and cognitive performance depends on water, which is essential for metabolism, temperature regulation, and numerous other physiological processes.[1] Accurate, precise, and reliable field measures are needed[1] to best assess an athlete's hydration status. Unfortunately, there is no "gold standard" for assessment of hydration status in the field setting[1,2]; however, several indices widely used in the clinical setting have been demonstrated to be accurate and valid. Selecting a hydration assessment technique for use in the field or clinical setting requires that the technique be easy to use, safe, portable, and inexpensive.[3] A commonly used technique to assess hydration status is weighing before and after activity to determine body mass change[1] based on fluid or sweat losses. Other accurate, reliable, and commonly used field measures are urine refractometry and urine color (Table 28-1).

Lopez RM, ed. *Quick Questions in Heat-Related Illness and Hydration: Expert Advice in Sports Medicine* (pp 151-156). © 2015 Taylor & Francis Group.

Table 28-1

Advantages and Disadvantages of Recommended (✓) and Not Recommended (×) Hydration Assessment Techniques

Recommended	Technique (Measure)	Advantages	Disadvantages
✓	Body mass change (% body mass loss)	• Easy; no training required • Equipment readily available • Inexpensive cost of analysis[3]	• Need euhydrated baseline • Must account for food/fluid consumption, urine and fecal losses[2]
✓	Handheld refractometer analog or digital (specific gravity)	• Digital versions reduce error • Inexpensive (~$150) and reusable • Requires minimal training	• Analog refractometers may introduce clinician error • May not accurately reflect hydration status* when used within a few minutes of exercise[1]
✓	Urine color (shades)	• Cost effective, easily accessible, portable • Easy to use • Requires negligible training	• Subjective interpretation is possible • Not as precise as refractometry
✓	Thirst perception (points)	• Efficient estimate • Useful educational tool	• Numerous factors may alter perception of thirst[1]
×	Urine reagent strips "dipstick" (specific gravity)	• Cost effective, easily accessible, portable • Easy to use	• Often unpredictable results[4] • Short shelf-life/expiration date • Must be stored properly
×	Bioelectrical impedance (body water)	• Quick and easy to administer • Equipment widely available (body composition scales)	• Various factors must be carefully controlled or results are not valid[2]

* All urine measures involve a time delay to allow kidney filtration and mixing with urine in the bladder

Body Mass Change

Because acute changes in body weight represent equal changes in hydration status,[2] body mass change is commonly used[1] to assess hydration. This technique is useful to assess dehydration that occurs over a period of several hours of activity (eg, long-distance endurance events) or repeated bouts of training or competition. When measuring body mass during relatively short periods of time (when an athlete's body is in caloric balance), body mass loss essentially equals water loss,[1,2] primarily from sweat. However, several limitations of this technique should be considered (see Table 28-1). In athletic settings, a baseline body mass is necessary and often difficult to obtain. Body mass fluctuates from day to day, requiring daily measurements to determine a stable normally hydrated baseline measure. Body mass measurements performed over several weeks cannot be interpreted as change in hydration because of the possible gain or loss of adipose tissue during extended periods.[1] Moreover, when an accurate normally hydrated baseline is unavailable or if weight is used repeatedly in a short period of time (days or weeks), chronic dehydration may go undetected. For more accuracy, this technique may require additional urine measures. In spite of these limitations, measuring hydration status through changes in body weight remains the best whole-body quantitative approach to be safely used in clinical/athletic settings.[2]

Urine Measures

URINE OSMOLALITY

Osmolality is the most widely used marker of hydration[2,3] in laboratory settings and is used as a reference standard of total solute content (all dissolved particles) in a known volume of fluid. This accuracy provides the best measurement of the kidney's concentrating ability.[1,3] Analysis requires an osmometer (relatively expensive and fragile) and a trained laboratory technician and is time consuming.[2] Because of these disadvantages, osmolality is typically reserved for laboratory analysis and is not widely used as a field measure of hydration status. As with all urinary hydration indices, these techniques may not accurately reflect hydration status when used within a few minutes of exercise.[1]

URINE SPECIFIC GRAVITY

Specific gravity refers to the density (mass per volume) of a sample compared with pure water. Any fluid denser than water has a specific gravity greater than 1.000,[1,3,4] with urine specific gravity exceeding 1.020 considered dehydration.[1,5] Although urine reagent strips (see Table 28-1) measuring specific gravity are cost effective, easily accessible, and easy to use,[4] a clinical refractometer is the preferred method of measuring urine specific gravity.[1,4] Research suggests that refractometry is a more sensitive indicator of hydration status and is more accurate than reagent strips (see Table 28-1), which often have unpredictable results.[4] Using an analog or digital handheld refractometer, specific gravity can be measured quickly and accurately. A few drops of a urine specimen are placed on the stage of the refractometer, which is then pointed toward a light source, allowing the clinician to determine specific gravity.[1] Digital refractometers are even quicker and easier to use as the tip of the refractometer "pen" is dipped into the sample, reducing time, supplies needed, and eliminating user error. Clinical refractometers are reusable and relatively inexpensive (< $199), so purchasing and using this device is a cost-effective, time-efficient, valid, and reliable measure of hydration status.

URINE COLOR

Urine color is an inexpensive clinical method for hydration measurement[4] that has been used with reasonable accuracy when laboratory analysis is not available or when a quick estimate of hydration is necessary.[1] Urine samples are subjectively compared with the urine color chart (Human Kinetics), and a score is obtained. Normal urine color is described as light yellow (score between 1 and 2 on the urine color chart); straw colored urine (score of 4) indicates mild hypohydration, whereas a urine color of brownish green (score > 6) indicates significant or severe hypohydration.[1] Anyone can determine urine color, although subjective interpretation is possible. Urine color does not offer the same precision and accuracy as urine specific gravity or osmolality[1]; however, it may be as good an indicator of hydration as urine osmolality.[2] Urine color is an effective measure of hydration status in clinical settings that do not require high precision.[1]

Bioelectrical Impedance

Electrical currents flowing through the human body (ie, from hands to feet) are resisted by body tissues and water. Measurements use this property to provide estimates of body composition, including body water.[1] Validation studies have verified that bioelectrical impedance may be reliable and valid with repeated measurements. However, a variety of factors may reduce the reliability and accuracy of this technique, including electrode site placement, skin temperature, skin blood flow, posture, recent fluid ingestion, composition of ingested fluids, exercise, and changes in plasma osmolality or plasma sodium concentration.[1] Bioelectrical impedance shows promise as a hydration-assessment technique, but it is not sufficiently accurate or reliable to measure hydration when posture or hydration states fluctuate. Therefore, as long as environmental and test subject factors are not controlled carefully, this hydration technique is not valid.[2]

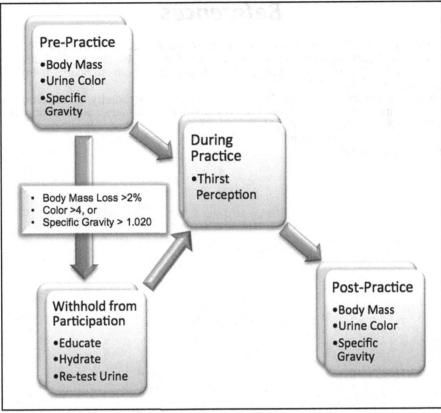

Figure 28-1. Recommended procedures for hydration testing.

Conclusion

Body water balance is a complex, dynamic, and ever-shifting process of maintaining hydration status to support sweat losses during exercise. It is important to appreciate the challenges in assessing hydration status, which are influenced by a variety of factors, such as water and sodium consumption and urinary and fecal losses.[3] Any hydration measure will be affected by the dynamic shifts of water throughout the body that are regulated by the renal and endocrine systems. Hydration assessment is a transitory moment in time, fluctuating throughout the day, and is affected by diet, physical activity, individual sweat rate, acclimatization, and environmental conditions. With these considerations in mind, using a variety of hydration assessment techniques depending on the setting and situation is necessary (Figure 28-1).

References

1. Armstrong LE. Hydration assessment techniques. *Nutr Rev.* 2005;63(6, pt 2):S40-S54.
2. Kavouras SA. Assessing hydration status. *Curr Opin Clin Nutr Metab Care.* 2002;5(5):519-524.
3. Armstrong LE. Assessing hydration status: the elusive gold standard. *J Am Coll Nutr.* 2007;26(5 suppl):S575-S584.
4. Eberman LE, Minton DM, Cleary MA. Comparison of refractometry, urine color, and urine reagent strips to urine osmolality for measurement of urinary concentration. *Athl Train Sports Health Care.* 2009;1(6):267-271.
5. Casa DJ, et al. National Athletic Trainers' Association position statement: exertional heat illnesses. *J Athl Train.* 2015;50.

HOW MUCH AND WHAT TYPES OF FLUID SHOULD BE CONSUMED BEFORE, DURING, AND AFTER EXERCISE OR TRAINING?

Lindsey E. Eberman, PhD, LAT, ATC

Just like all difficult questions, there is no easy answer to this age-old question. Fluid replacement needs during exercise vary among individuals and, unfortunately, there is no one-size-fits-all answer. The best global recommendations are to drink regularly before, during, and after exercise in order to match your losses with your gains (Table 29-1). Environmental conditions, equipment considerations, heat acclimatization, and intensity and length of exercise heavily affect sweat rate. Furthermore, the taste and temperature of a fluid can affect our willingness to consume it. So, let's get into some specifics.

Although there are 3 commonly used and effective clinical hydration measurements (body mass loss, urine specific gravity, and urine color),[1] knowing one's own sweat rate will aid in the development of an individualized fluid replacement plan.

Lopez RM, ed. *Quick Questions in Heat-Related Illness and Hydration: Expert Advice in Sports Medicine* (pp 157-160).
© 2015 Taylor & Francis Group.

Table 29-1	
Recommendations for Fluid Replacement Before, During, and After Exercise	
	Recommendation
Before	• Large bolus of water (500 to 600 mL) 2 to 3 hours before exercise • 200 to 300 mL within 10 to 20 minutes before exercise
During	• Use an individualized fluid replacement plan • Match losses with gains using the sweat rate calculation
After	• Restrict athlete from participation unless body mass is within 2% of baseline • Use both fluid and food to return body water and electrolyte balance to pre-exercise levels

$$\text{Sweat Rate} = \frac{(\text{Pre-Exercise Body Weight [kg]} - \text{Post-Exercise Body Weight [kg]} + \text{Fluid Intake [L]} - \text{Urine Volume [L]})^*}{\text{Time [hours]}}$$

*To avoid urine collection, a pre-exercise body weight after voiding and post-exercise body weight before voiding can make the calculation easier.

Environmental conditions can increase the risk for hypohydration, and as such, the incidence of heat-related illnesses. In addition, the restrictions of protective equipment to allow for evaporative cooling can stifle the body's ability to thermoregulate through sweating. Therefore, when calculating sweat rate, we need to consider the environment and equipment to accurately anticipate fluid replacement needs in the given conditions in which we intend to exercise.

Because sport exercise and physical training often vary greatly in length and intensity, it is difficult to pinpoint a total volume to consume during activity. The longer one exercises, the lower the intensity of the exercise and, based on basic physiological principles, the less risk of exertional heat illness. Therefore, the increased risk for heat illness often occurs during shorter, more intense bouts of exercise. Although hypohydration is not always associated with heat illness in these cases, repeated bouts of intense exercise without adequate fluid replacement can increase this risk. As such, fluid replacement following exercise, specifically in several, smaller volumes within 6 hours following exercise, can help to prevent fluid depletion.[1]

Once sweat rate is calculated, athletes can easily match fluid volume intake to output. Depending on the type of exercise, intensity, and environmental conditions, calculating an average sweat rate across 2 to 3 days of similar conditions is recommended to accurately represent losses during exercise.

Replacement can also be influenced by the temperature and taste of fluid. Historical research has suggested that a carbohydrate electrolyte solution or juice is more palatable and will increase the likelihood of consumption, resulting in a positive fluid balance.[2] In addition, newer findings have confirmed that cooler temperatures can prevent hypohydration; a cold (10°C), carbohydrate-electrolyte solution is most favorable for consumption and weight retention compared with plain water and moderate-temperature beverages.[3] We also know that carbohydrate-electrolyte solutions are less likely to result in fullness compared with other beverages.[3]

Generally speaking, athletes of varying competition levels fail to adequately replace fluids and nutrients prior to, during, and after exercise.[1] Fluid, however, is not the only considerable loss during exercise. Carbohydrates and electrolytes are necessary as the body continues to fight for homeostasis, particularly through exercise. A 6% carbohydrate solution is favorable for gastric emptying and absorption.[4] The consumption of 60 to 80 g of carbohydrate per hour is effective at delaying fatigue and staving off performance degradation and perceived exertion during vigorous exercise.[1] In addition, guidelines for sodium replacement suggest adding 0.7 to 1.2 g/L of sodium to fluid during exercise and recovery to stimulate thirst, increase voluntary fluid intake, enhance glucose and water intestinal absorption, and optimize fluid balance.[1]

Clinically, the bottom line is that an individualized fluid replacement plan is best. If at all possible, athletes should match fluid intake to fluid losses using a calculated sweat rate, and be wary of carbohydrate and electrolyte losses, particularly in endurance exercises. Between exercise sessions, athletes should monitor body weight losses and attempt to replace fluid lost before the next exercise session (1 kg = 1 L). In cases where clinicians are overburdened with a large volume of patients, at minimum, athletes that are at risk for hypohydration or heat illness should be identified. In addition, teaching athletes about hydration practices, including measuring their own sweat rate, can ameliorate the task to providing individualized plans for several patients.

A comparative example of typical sweat rate calculations for 2 athletes is on page 160. Consider that both are likely exercising in similar environmental conditions, yet one is wearing protective equipment. Further, one is likely exercising more intensely for a shorter period of time, yet both yield similar sweat rates.

Football lineman
- 21 years old
- Body mass before exercise: 136.1 kg (300 lb)
- Exercises for 150 minutes (2.5 h)
- Body mass after exercise: 132.1 kg (291.2 lb)
- 136.1 − 132.1 kg = (4 / 136.1 kg)*100 = 2.9% body mass lost
- Fluid consumed: 3 L
- Fluid excreted: 0.25 L
- $\dfrac{(136.1\,kg - 132.1\,kg + 3\,L - 0.25\,L)}{2.5\,h} = 2.7\,L/hr$

Cross-country runner
- 14 years old
- Body mass before exercise: 69.9 kg (154 lb)
- Exercises for 60 minutes (1 h)
- Body mass after exercise: 68.4 kg (151 lb)
- 69.9 − 68.4 kg = (1.5 / 69.9 kg)*100 = 2.0% body mass lost
- Fluid consumed: 0.5 L
- Fluid excreted: 0 L
- $\dfrac{(69.9\,kg - 68.4\,kg + 0.5\,L - 0\,L)}{1\,h} = 2\,L/hr$

In these examples, the resultant clinical practice would be to ensure that these athletes adequately replace these fluids during physical activity (replacing the 2 to 2.7 L for every 1 h of exercise). In the event that these fluids are not matched, replacing fluid and electrolytes through drink and food between practices is necessary. This should include educating athletes about what body mass loss means and how to monitor their own progress toward returning to baseline levels. Losses beyond 2% have negative impacts on performance and, moreover, lead to increased risk for heat illness. Athletes exceeding 2% body mass loss should be restricted from consecutive practices until fluid has been replaced. As athletes approach consecutive practices, a large bolus of water (500 to 600 mL) 2 to 3 hours before and again 200 to 300 mL within 10 to 20 minutes prior to exercise can also help to ensure proper pre-exercise hydration.[5]

References

1. Casa DJ, Clarkson PM, Roberts WO. American College of Sports Medicine roundtable on hydration and physical activity: consensus statements. *Curr Sports Med Rep.* 2005;4:115-127.
2. Maughan RJ, Leiper JB. Post-exercise rehydration in man: effects of voluntary intake on four different beverages. *Med Sci Sports Exerc.* 1993;25:1358-1364.
3. Park SG, Bae YJ, Lee YS, Kiim BJ. Effects of rehydration fluid temperature and composition on body weight retention upon voluntary drinking following exercise-induced dehydration. *Nutr Res Pract.* 2012;6:126-131.
4. Murray R, Bartoli WP, Eddy DE, Horn MK. Gastric emptying and plasma deuterium accumulation following ingestion of water and two carbohydrate-electrolyte beverages. *Int J Sports Nutr.* 1997;7:144-153.
5. Casa DJ, Armstrong LE, Hillman SK, et al. National Athletic Trainers' Association position statement: fluid replacement for athletes. *J Athl Train.* 2000;35(2):212-224.

HOW DOES ONE CALCULATE SWEAT RATE AND SWEAT SODIUM LOSSES IN AN ATHLETE, AND HOW MUCH OF THE WEIGHT LOSS DUE TO SWEATING SHOULD BE REPLACED BEFORE THE NEXT PRACTICE OR EVENT?

Nicole E. Moyen, MS, CSCS and Matthew S. Ganio, PhD

Inadequate replacement of sweat and electrolytes lost during exercise can impair performance; therefore, a hydration plan should be incorporated that is tailored to each individual's fluid balance needs during exercise.[1] This section provides ways to calculate sweat rate and electrolyte losses during exercise to develop an accurate, individualized fluid replacement plan to optimize performance.

Water Losses Through Sweat

Heat loss during exercise primarily occurs through sweat evaporation. Increased body temperature (via exercise or hot environments) elevates sweat rate (ie, sweat output per minute or hour). Since sweat rates widely vary (average 1 to 2 L·h⁻¹, but can be 3 to 4 L·h⁻¹), it is important to calculate each individual's sweat rate.[1]

As body temperature increases, it reaches a temperature where sweating begins (ie, the sweat threshold/onset). Sweat rate continues to increase as body temperature rises; this change in sweat rate per degree increase in body temperature is

Lopez RM, ed. *Quick Questions in Heat-Related Illness and Hydration: Expert Advice in Sports Medicine* (pp 161-165). © 2015 Taylor & Francis Group.

Table 30-1

Internal and External Factors Altering Sweat Parameters

	Sweat Rate	Sweat Threshold[a]	Sweat Sensitivity[b]	Sweat Electrolyte Concentration
Sex	males > females	↔	↔	↔
Aging[c]	↓	↑	↓	↔
Heat acclimatization	↑	↓	↑	↓
Improved aerobic fitness	↑	↓	↑	↓
Hot/humid climates	↑	↔	↔	↑
Sport uniform/ protective clothing[d]	↑	unknown	unknown	↔
Dehydration	↓	↑	↓	↑

Arrows indicate whether the sweat rate, sweat threshold, sweat sensitivity, and sweat electrolyte concentrations increase (↑), decrease (↓), or remain unchanged (↔) based on the factors in the first column. Information compiled from Sawka et al[1] and Taylor et al.[2]

[a] Refers to the body temperature when sweating begins. Increased threshold/onset means sweating begins at a higher body temperature, delaying evaporative heat loss.

[b] Refers to the sweat output per degree increase in body temperature. Increased sensitivity means more sweat will be secreted per degree increase in body temperature, allowing for greater evaporative heat loss.

[c] Refers to those >35 to 40 years.

[d] Refers to sport gear that covers a large portion of the body surface area thereby restricting evaporative heat loss and increasing core temperature (eg, football uniform).

called sweat sensitivity. The sweat threshold, sensitivity, and overall sweat rate vary between and within individuals based on several different individual (ie, internal and external) factors. Internal factors affecting sweating include sex, age, aerobic fitness, hydration status, and acclimatization. External factors include environmental conditions and type of sport uniform.[1,2] Table 30-1 shows factors that modify sweat parameters; these factors should be considered when evaluating an athlete. It is important for practitioners to re-evaluate athletes throughout the season because changes in these factors (eg, fitness, environmental conditions, heat acclimatization) will alter sweat rate and sweat electrolyte concentrations.

The simplest, most practical way to determine sweat rate is to use body mass changes before and after exercise. Prior to exercise, the athlete should empty his or her bladder and then obtain a nude body mass. Fluids consumed or urine produced during exercise should be measured and accounted for. After exercise, the athlete should wipe off all sweat before weighing nude again. Sweat rate is calculated as follows (body mass is in kilograms; fluid consumed and urine produced is in liters; time is in hours)[1,3]:

$$\text{Sweat rate } (L \cdot h^{-1}) = [(\text{mass pre} - \text{mass post}) + \text{fluid consumed} - \text{urine produced}] \div \text{time}$$

Electrolyte Losses Through Sweat

Sweat mostly consists of water (99.0% to 99.5%) but also contains electrolytes essential to basic physiological function. The primary sweat electrolytes are sodium (~10 to 70 mmol·L^{-1} or mEq·L^{-1}), chloride (~5 to 60 mmol·L^{-1} or mEq·L^{-1}), and potassium (~3 to 15 mmol·L^{-1} or mEq·L^{-1}).[1] Sweat electrolyte concentrations vary between individuals and settings (see Table 30-1), hence the importance of obtaining individualized values.

Knowledge of sweat electrolyte concentrations is most valuable and applicable when combined with sweat rate (see above). The more an individual sweats, the more absolute electrolyte losses occur. Typically, though, sweat rates of 1 to 2 L·h^{-1} result in sodium and chloride losses of less than ~1.6 g·L^{-1} and ~2.1 g·L^{-1}, respectively.

To measure sweat electrolyte losses, a representative sweat sample must be collected and analyzed. Procedures for sweat collection vary based on time, equipment, money, and expertise. The whole-body rinse technique is the most valid method to evaluate whole-body sweat electrolyte losses,[3] but the regional sweat patch technique can be used as a feasible and practical alternative for clinicians.[4]

The following procedures give an overview of the whole-body rinse technique (for more detailed methods, see Armstrong et al[3]):

1. The athlete's body and clothes are washed with deionized water before exercise.

2. The athlete's pre-exercise body mass (wearing electrolyte-free clothing) is obtained.

3. The athlete exercises for 30 to 60 minutes in a warm environment without consuming fluids.

4. During exercise, the athlete wipes all sweat with towels.

5. A post-exercise body mass (clothing still on) is obtained.

6. Approximately 2 L of distilled water is poured over the athlete while rinsing/scrubbing the entire body to ensure that all sweat enters the tub.

7. All towels/clothing are placed in the rinse water and mixed together to ensure that all electrolytes are extracted.

8. A small sample of tub water is obtained and analyzed for sodium and chloride concentrations. The following equation gives the electrolyte concentrations ([E]) per liter of sweat (mmol·L^{-1}).

$$[E] = [([E] \text{ obtained via the analyzer}) \cdot \text{distilled water volume used (L)}]$$
$$\div (\text{Pre body mass (kg)} - \text{Post body mass (kg)})$$

The regional sweat patch technique has the same goal: inducing sweating and collecting it for analysis via "sweat patches" placed on the skin during exercise. Because sweat rate and electrolyte concentrations vary across the body, samples from multiple sites are needed; the forearm, superior scapula, upper chest, forehead, and anterior midthigh are most commonly used. Before application, each site is cleaned with distilled water, and the patch is weighed. As the individual exercises, the patch collects sweat and is removed once saturated. The patch is weighed again, placed in a test tube, and centrifuged to extract the sweat. The regression equation, which follows, estimates sweat electrolyte concentrations.[4]

Estimate of sweat

$$\text{electrolyte concentrations} = (0.07[E]_{FH} \cdot SR_{FH} + 0.36[E]_{TR} \cdot SR_{TR} +$$
$$0.13[E]_{FA} \cdot SR_{FA} + 0.32[E]_{T} \cdot SR_{T}) \div$$
$$(0.07 \cdot SR_{FH} + 0.36 \cdot SR_{TR} + 0.13 \cdot SR_{FA} + 0.32 \cdot SR_{T})$$

where SR is local sweat rate (mg·min^{-1}·cm^{-2}), calculated by changes in the patch weight, size of the patch, and length of time on the site. (FH is forehead; TR is trunk, which is the superior scapula and upper chest averaged; FA is forearm; T is anterior midthigh.)

Although this procedure is more practical than the whole-body rinse technique, it can sometimes overestimate sweat electrolyte concentrations.

Replacing Water and Electrolyte Losses

Ideally, athletes replace all water and electrolytes lost while exercising. However, most settings are not conducive to this and/or the amount to be replaced is unknown. Therefore, after exercise athletes need to determine their water/electrolyte deficiencies and replace those losses. Accounting for urine produced, body mass change from pre- to post-exercise usually indicates fluids lost during exercise (eg, if the athlete weighs 1 kg less after exercise, he or she has not replaced 1 L of fluid). However, simply drinking 1 L of fluid after exercise does not necessarily replace the kilogram of fluid lost. If the athlete quickly drinks 1 L of water, the body increases urine production to prevent dilution of blood concentrations, and consequently net fluid retention will be less than 1 L. Thus, after exercise, it is recommended that athletes slowly drink ~20 oz per pound (1.5 L per kilogram) of body mass lost during exercise. The exact amount depends on other factors such as food ingested and sodium content in beverages consumed.

Sodium content of the recovery drink largely influences fluid retention. Replacing 150% to 200% of sweat losses with drinks containing high sodium (~1.3 $g \cdot L^{-1}$) results in optimal fluid and sodium retention compared with consuming lower sodium (~0.5 $g \cdot L^{-1}$) drinks; consuming greater volumes of low sodium drinks after exercise only increases urination, not fluid retention.[5] Therefore, rehydrating with drinks containing high concentrations of sodium (~1 $g \cdot L^{-1}$) will increase fluid retention and help the athlete achieve adequate hydration.

Conclusion

Creating an optimal hydration plan requires calculating sweat rate several times throughout the year to account for the various factors affecting sweat rate. The easiest way to measure sweat rate is to obtain nude body mass measurements before and after exercise, accounting for fluid consumed and urine produced. Electrolyte losses should also be calculated and replaced by foods/fluids after exercise. Athletes should strive to replace fluids lost by consuming drinks containing high concentrations of sodium immediately after exercise to facilitate rehydration and recovery.

References

1. Sawka MN, Burke LM, Eichner ER, Maughan RJ, Montain SJ, Stachenfeld NS. American college of sports medicine position stand: exercise and fluid replacement. *Med Sci Sports Exerc.* 2007;39(2):377-390.
2. Taylor NA, Machado-Moreira CA. Regional variations in transepidermal water loss, eccrine sweat gland density, sweat secretion rates and electrolyte composition in resting and exercising humans. *Extreme Physiol Med.* 2013;2(1):1-30.
3. Armstrong L, Casa D. Methods to evaluate electrolyte and water turnover of athletes. *Athletic Training & Sports Health Care.* 2009;1:169-179.
4. Baker LB, Stofan JR, Hamilton AA, Horswill CA. Comparison of regional patch collection vs whole body washdown for measuring sweat sodium and potassium loss during exercise. *J Appl Physiol.* 2009;107(3):887-895.
5. Shirreffs SM, Taylor AJ, Leiper JB, Maughan RJ. Post-exercise rehydration in man: effects of volume consumed and drink sodium content. *Med Sci Sports Exerc.* 1996;28(10):1260-1271.

Is Intravenous Fluid Superior to Oral Fluid Rehydration When Replacing Fluid Losses Due to Exercise?

Brendon P. McDermott, PhD, ATC

Many athletes and recreational exercisers complete exercise in a state of hypohydration, or decreased body water content. The ideal goal before, during, and following exercise should be to maintain a state of euhydration, or ideal body water.[1] This is rarely achieved. Most athletes begin exercise with less than ideal water content, never mind those exercising recreationally. While most athletes begin exercise hypohydrated, they do a pretty good job during exercise of replacing, on average, about 75% of fluid losses. However, this maintains the hypohydrated state that was present at the onset of exercise. So, after exercise, it is important to remedy the hypohydration and get back to, or at least achieve, euhydration. Replacing fluids after exercise will help replenish losses and expedite recovery.[2]

Intravenous (IV) fluids are commonly used as an efficient avenue to replace fluids in sports medicine. Most often, IV fluid administration is used to correct dehydration and severe exercise-associated muscle cramping. In the past 10 years or so, IV fluid usage has increased. It is now used for prevention of dehydration, treatment of illness, as a means to facilitate recovery when rest breaks are short (halftime, stage race, etc), and to improve performance.

Lopez RM, ed. *Quick Questions in Heat-Related Illness and Hydration: Expert Advice in Sports Medicine* (pp 167-170).
© 2015 Taylor & Francis Group.

Administration of IV fluids is sometimes thought of as a rite of passage in the locker room. Some athletes can probably be heard bragging about how bad their dehydration was, and that they required an IV. IV fluids are often overused where there is little regulation against their use. Anecdotally, some sports medicine professionals have more than 10 L in a cooler for a field hockey practice during the summer. Also, some high schools use preventive IV fluids for football players prior to and/or during halftime to avoid dehydration and exercise-associated muscle cramping. However, some administrative bodies (International Olympic Committee, World Anti-Doping Agency) have banned the use of IV fluids because of the chance that it offers an unfair advantage over the competition. This is in cases where an underlying illness, beyond simple exercise dehydration, is not present. Interestingly, neither banning IV fluids nor allowing them without medical necessity is supported by evidence-based medicine at this point.

What we do know about IV fluids is that they rapidly restore plasma volume levels and blood osmolality.[2-4] This is unquestioned as a short-term and rapid advantage that seems to restore homeostasis. However, rehydration is more complicated than the rate of fluid delivery into the body's vasculature. Contrary to popular belief, IV fluids have not shown further advantage over oral fluid intake to correct exercise dehydration beyond rapid plasma volume expansion. IV fluids offer only short-term plasma expansion even when fluid tonicity differences exist (eg, normal saline IV versus one-half normal saline).[5] This is important to consider because oral fluids are intolerable beyond a concentration of one-half normal saline, but the IV route allows higher concentrations. When matched or varied concentrations were given in trials comparing IV and oral fluids, no difference between oral and IV fluid rehydration in outcomes related to hemodynamic and cardiovascular stress (respiratory rate, cardiac output, skin blood flow, or oxygen uptake) were identified.[3,4] The expedient delivery of IV fluids allows a faster fluid expansion, but offers no advantage in terms of retaining those fluids. The oral route of fluid ingestion causes a cascade of events as a result of mouth wetting and the act of swallowing. This is initiated as part of the oropharyngeal reflex. Further, stress hormone responses and exercise in the heat following rehydration using both methods demonstrates virtually no differences between IV and oral fluids.[3,4]

For some variables, simultaneous stimulation of oropharyngeal reflexes and rapid plasma volume expansion via IV may offer benefits beyond those identified with a single method of rehydration following exercise.[4] This offers some evidence in support of clinicians who offer oral fluids in conjunction with IV when an IV is necessary. This combination administration may speed recovery further than either oral or IV rehydration alone.[2]

There is no clear-cut answer to the question at hand, it seems. Using IV fluids offers some expediency, while oral fluids are more natural for the body and help

Table 31-1

Comparison of Responses Between Intravenous and Oral Fluid Rehydration

	Intravenous Fluids	Oral Fluids	Combination of Oral and IV Fluids
Acute plasma volume expansion (30 min)	✓+		✓
Thirst alleviation		✓+	✓
Subsequent athletic performance	=	=	Not tested
Heart rate recovery	=	=	=
Blood pressure recovery	=	=	✓
Plasma volume restoration (60 min)	=	=	=
Stress hormone recovery	=	=	=
Thermoregulation (heat tolerance)	=	=	=

✓+, Better than all others; ✓, Better than ( ) and (=); =, no differences.

restore physiology from within (Table 31-1). In terms of practicing ethical sports medicine, health care professionals should use caution when using IV rehydration. We should take into consideration the risk:benefit ratio and make an ethical decision and establish protocols on the best available recommendations to date. Those who use IV fluids on demand because athletes do not take care of themselves run the risk of overusing IV fluids, as word spreads quickly on teams. Health care professionals should work together to establish good hydration practices and document good reasons for IV usage prior to the season. There are risks associated with administering an IV. There is documentation of bruising, infection, and vasovagal syncope as the most common risk factors with IV usage.

There are times when dehydrated patients cannot tolerate oral fluids. They may be suffering from multiple muscle group intense cramping, or they may be vomiting.[1] In some cases oral fluids will be rejected by patients, representing a failure in treatment. When a patient cannot tolerate oral fluids for these reasons, and dehydration is confirmed, IV fluids are the gold standard in treatment. At this point, IV fluids should be provided until symptoms are minimized and the patient can tolerate oral fluids again. In the case of muscle cramping, there is plenty of anecdotal evidence that rapid IV saline administration reduces muscle cramping quickly (within minutes). Interesting to note is that it has yet to be determined why this works with muscle cramping. Is it the sodium restoration? Is it the fluid replacement? The truth is, we don't really know.

Last, consider the scenario of a case of exertional hyponatremia. The signs and symptoms of low blood sodium levels parallel those of dehydration (overall fatigue, dizziness, nausea, etc). A patient who has exertional hyponatremia does not benefit from normal saline IV administration and actually could worsen because of it. In some cases where dehydration was assumed, the patient was treated with IV fluids, and death from hyponatremia occurred. Medical tents at distance events where hyponatremia is commonly seen have mandated blood-sodium assessment prior to IV administration. Health care professionals should consider this as a means of preventing unwarranted worsening of hyponatremia because the diagnosis is assumed to be dehydration. We should confirm a diagnosis of dehydration with normal blood sodium levels prior to administering IV fluids to patients. This is another reason why, perhaps, IV fluids ought to be used with caution and only in certain circumstances. And, when they are required, the addition of oral fluids simultaneously seems to maximize outcomes.

References

1. Casa DJ, Armstrong LE, Hillman SK, et al. National athletic trainers' association position statement: fluid replacement for athletes. *J Athl Train.* 2000;35(2):212-234.
2. McDermott BP, Casa DJ, Lee EC, et al. The influence of rehydration mode after exercise dehydration on cardiovascular function. *J Strength Cond Res.* 2013;27(8):2086-2095.
3. Casa DJ, Ganio MS, Lopez RM, McDermott BP, Armstrong LE, Maresh CM. Intravenous versus oral rehydration: physiological, performance and legal considerations. *Curr Sports Med Rep.* 2008;7(4):S41-S49.
4. McDermott BP, Casa DJ, Lee E, et al. Thermoregulation and stress hormone recovery after exercise dehydration: comparison of rehydration methods. *J Athl Train.* 2013;48(6):725-733.
5. Kenefick RW, Maresh CM, Armstrong LE, Riebe D, Echegaray ME, Castellani JW. Rehydration with fluid of varying tonicities: effects on fluid regulatory hormones and exercise performance in the heat. *J Appl Physiol.* 2007;102(5):1899-1905.

SHOULD SODIUM (VIA FOODS, SALT TABLETS, OR PICKLE JUICE) BE CONSUMED PRIOR TO OR DURING ENDURANCE ACTIVITIES FOR THE PREVENTION OF EXERTIONAL HEAT ILLNESS?

J. Luke Pryor, MS, ATC, CSCS and Deanna M. Dempsey, MS

It is well established that maintaining hydration is integral in preventing exertional heat illnesses (EHI).[1,2] Sodium plays a vital role in the ability of the human body to maintain a hydrated state due to the water retention capabilities of sodium. Dramatic reductions in both sodium and water balance can occur during endurance activities as a result of sweat sodium and fluid losses. Thus, endurance athletes must take precautionary measures to maintain sodium and water balance prior to and during exercise to prevent exertional heat injury.

A wide range of sweat rates and sodium concentrations has been reported, from 0.5 to well over 2.5 L/h (1 to 5 lb) and salt (NaCl) losses of 0.8 to 4.0 g/L[2]. Over the course of a 4-hour marathon, a runner with a sweat rate and sodium concentration of 2.0 L/h and 2.0 g/L, respectively, could lose 16 lb of water and 8.0 g of salt. A sodium (and fluid) deficiency is entirely possible, particularly when intake does not match losses. Several factors influence sweat production and composition, including body mass and composition, exercise duration and intensity, nutrition, clothing, heat acclimatization status, heredity, hydration level, environmental conditions, sport and position, and fitness level.[1,2] Competing

Lopez RM, ed. *Quick Questions in Heat-Related Illness and Hydration: Expert Advice in Sports Medicine* (pp 171-176). © 2015 Taylor & Francis Group.

and/or training at high intensities, over prolonged periods, on consecutive days, multiple times per day, or during the initial days of heat exposure increase the risk of sodium and fluid deficiency. In these scenarios, supplemental sodium (and fluid) intake matched to the amount lost is suggested by both the American College of Sports Medicine and National Athletic Trainers' Association for the prevention of EHI.[1,2]

This section will highlight the importance and briefly discuss the role of sodium (and fluid) in EHI, including exertional heat cramps, exhaustion, and stroke. Although exercise-associated hyponatremia is not classified as an EHI, the central role of sodium in its etiology warrants discussion herein.

Exertional Heat Cramps

While controversial, some evidence suggests that sodium supplementation may prevent muscle cramps. Two primary types of muscular cramps characterized by their symptoms have been identified. First, exercise-associated muscle cramps (EAMC) are localized and prompted by an overloaded neuromuscular system and/or fatigued muscle that can be resolved by passive stretching and massage. Emerging evidence suggests that for these types of muscle cramps sodium supplementation has little to no effect.[3] By comparison, exertional heat cramps are usually bilateral and can affect a single or several muscle groups. Extensive sweating over prolonged periods can lead to sweat-induced whole body exchangeable sodium and fluid deficit, which has been implicated in exertional heat cramps.[4] Sodium deficits in endurance athletes have been documented in as little as 45 minutes of high intensity exercise but usually occur over prolonged races (eg, triathlons) or over several days as sweat sodium losses exceed dietary intake (eg, consecutive days of football or soccer practice). Thus, the insidious development of heat cramps may be surprising to athletes given that they didn't previously incur any problems under similar circumstances.

The prevention of exertional heat cramps involves the maintenance of sodium and fluid balance.[4] Exploring methods to diminish dramatic perturbations in sodium and fluid balance is recommended.[1,2,4] This is particularly important during prolonged exercise in hot, humid conditions, when sodium and fluid losses can be high.

Heat Exhaustion and Exertional Heat Stroke

Heat exhaustion as a result of salt depletion occurs during prolonged events in hot, humid environments in athletes who have high sweat rates and who replace fluid losses with hypotonic solutions. For this type of heat exhaustion, matching sodium and fluid intake to losses is warranted. The link between sodium deficiency and heat stroke has not been extensively studied because of the ethical limitations of inducing exertional heat stroke in humans. However, it stands to reason that maintaining sodium balance indirectly contributes to preventing heat stroke by maintaining euhydration, which subsequently reduces cardiovascular and thermoregulatory strain.

Exercise-Associated Hyponatremia

Although exercise-associated hyponatremia is not a heat illness, it merits discussion here because of the role of sodium in this condition. Exercise-associated hyponatremia is characterized by low serum sodium levels (< 130 mmol/L) and usually occurs during long or ultra endurance races that take place in the heat. Two, often synergistic, mechanisms explain hyponatremia: overdrinking hypotonic fluids such as water (termed *water intoxication*) and sweat sodium losses not being adequately replaced.[1] Hyponatremia can be prevented by consuming high-sodium–containing fluids and foods to replace losses (Table 32-1).

Strategies to Minimize Exertional Heat Illnesses Through Sodium Consumption

There is no optimal fluid and sodium intake that is recommended for all athletes. It is recommended that periodic assessments of both sweat rate and sodium losses be performed to optimize individualized diet and hydration plans before and during sports. Although most athletes following a Western diet consume enough sodium to meet losses, except during the initial days of heat exposure and training, assessment of sodium and fluid losses during exercise is warranted to minimize EHI risk and sustain performance.

Sodium losses from sweat are best determined using the whole-body rinse down technique and an electrolyte analyzer. If an electrolyte analyzer is not feasible, some degree of whether an athlete is a "salty sweater" can be determined by having the athlete wear a black shirt while exercising for 30 minutes to 1 hour at race pace (Figure 32-1). Any accumulation of white particulate (especially around the armpits, chest, and upper back) indicates a salty sweater. Fluid losses via sweating are determined by calculating the difference between pre- and post-exercise body mass.

Generally, for athletes at risk for sodium deficiency, matching sodium intake to losses can be achieved by salting foods consumed within their normal balanced

Table 32-1

Sodium and Macronutrient Content in Common Foods Consumed Prior to or During Endurance Events

	Serving Size	Calories	Protein	Fat	CHO	Sodium
Pickle juice	1 oz	0	0 g	0 g	0 g	820 mg
Bouillon broth	1 oz	3	0 g	0.6 g	0 g	600 mg
Plain bagel	1	270	11 g	2 g	53 g	470 mg
Pretzel twists	17 pretzels	110	2 g	1 g	23 g	450 mg
Cheddar cheese	1/2 cup	265	16 g	22 g	1 g	410 mg
Gatorade Endurance Formula	8 oz	50	0 g	0 g	14 g	200 mg
Chocolate Powerbar	1 bar	240	8 g	3 g	45 g	200 mg
Saltine crackers	5 crackers	70	1 g	12 g	15 g	150 mg
Yellow mustard	1 tbsp	0	0 g	0 g	0 g	165 mg
Jif (JM Smucker Co) regular creamy peanut butter	2 tbsp	183	7 g	16 g	8 g	135 mg
GU Energy Gel	1 package	100	0 g	2 g	20 g	125 mg
Salted almonds	28 nuts	180	6 g	16 g	5 g	120 mg
Gatorade G2	8 oz	50	0 g	0 g	14 g	110 mg
Gatorade Energy Chews	6 chews	100	0 g	0 g	25 g	55 mg
Large banana	136 g	121	1 g	0 g	31 g	1 mg

Abbreviation: CHO, carbohydrate.

diet. Fluid-electrolyte beverages (eg, Gatorade) are popular drinks that claim to provide adequate electrolyte replacement for athletes. However, these beverages contain only a small amount of salt (0.1 to 0.3 g salt per 20 oz) and cannot fully replace sodium losses during prolonged endurance events. Adding ¼ to

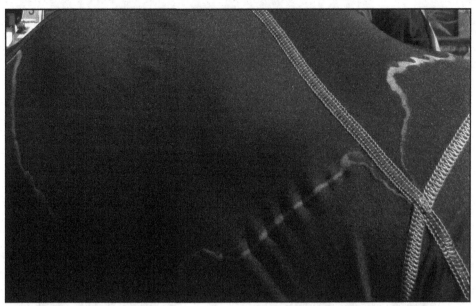

Figure 32-1. Salt particulate observed on a black shirt after a half marathon race in April. Evidence of a salty sweater.

½ teaspoons of table salt per 20 ounces of sports drink improves sodium delivery. If taste is an issue, add ½ teaspoon of salt to 32 ounces. Some individuals choose to eat pickles or drink pickle juice to increase sodium consumption (Figure 32-2). Ingesting whole salt tablets is not recommended as they create a large osmotic gradient in the gut, potentially leading to gastrointestinal stress. It is important to note that new hydration, sodium supplementation, and/or food plans should be practiced prior to implementation in competitions.

Conclusion

The current scientific evidence suggests that sodium supplementation matched to losses with adequate fluid ingestion assists in the prevention of EHI. Except during the initial days of heat exposure and training, supplemental sodium is not necessary, as dietary sodium covers sweat losses in the typical American diet. When increasing dietary sodium intake to match sweat losses, caution should be taken in individuals who are salt sensitive, hypertensive, or on a low-sodium diet for medical purposes. A physician consultation is recommended in this instance.

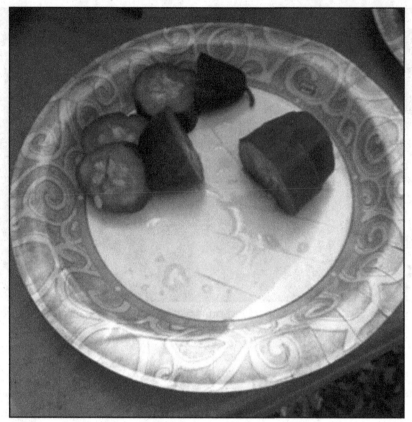

Figure 32-2. Pickles available to runners during a 50-km endurance trail race.

References

1. Casa DJ, et al. National Athletic Trainers' Association position statement: exertional heat illnesses. *J Athl Train*. 2015;50.
2. Armstrong LE, Casa DJ, Millard-Stafford M, et al. Exertional heat illness during training and competition. *Med Sci Sports Exer*. 2007;39(3):556-572.
3. Minetto MA, Holobar A, Botter A, Farina D. Origin and development of muscle cramps. *Exer Sport Sci Rev*. 2013;41(1):3-10.
4. Bergeron MF. Muscle cramps during exercise: is it fatigue or electrolyte deficit? *Curr Sports Med Rep*. 2008;7(4):S50-S55.

HOW LONG SHOULD AN ATHLETIC TRAINER MONITOR PRE- AND POST-PRACTICE WEIGH-INS?

Mike D. Ryan, PT, ATC, CES, PES

The dangers of exertional heat illness (EHI) are well documented. The sports medicine field has witnessed far too many deaths related to heat illness involving youth, high school, collegiate, and professional athletes. Multiple factors contribute to EHI. The main categories for these factors include environmental, clothing/equipment, physiological, and the activity itself. It is extremely important to note that with the right tools and preparation, clinicians can take several steps to prevent EHI. Athletic trainers around the world have been the driving force to combat EHI for athletes, young and old.

One of the key steps to monitoring athletes, in the effort to minimize their risk for heat illness, is to weigh athletes both before and immediately after their activities. This process of weighing players in and out is a simple and effective way to determine how much weight an athlete has lost during his or her activity. The benefits of pre- and post-exercise weigh-ins are numerous and cannot be overemphasized. A key step to preventing human illness is early intervention. Knowing if an athlete has lost 2% or higher of his or her body weight is very important for an athletic trainer and for the athlete him- or herself to avoid complications related to

Lopez RM, ed. *Quick Questions in Heat-Related Illness and Hydration: Expert Advice in Sports Medicine* (pp 177-181).
© 2015 Taylor & Francis Group.

dehydration. This information tells the athlete whether or not fluid intake matched sweat losses during a given bout of exercise. It also allows the clinician an opportunity to educate athletes and ensure they are rehydrating before the next practice or athletic event. Table 33-1 is a sample weight chart that can be used to identify athletes who may be at risk of EHI.

Tips to Maximize Effectiveness of the Weigh-In/-Out

- Clothing: The individual should consistently wear only a dry shirt and shorts for both the pre- and post-exercise weigh-ins. Variations in clothing will alter the weights and reduce the accuracy of the exact number of pounds lost during a game, practice, or conditioning session.
- Timing: The weigh-ins should take place immediately before and immediately after the workout/game to properly monitor the athlete's weight. If, after a practice the athlete is allowed to urinate or consume fluids prior to obtaining the body weight measurement, the numbers will reflect this.
- Documentation: It is beneficial to have a staff member available to see the weight and document it accordingly, thus eliminating the potential for athletes to adjust the numbers.
- Education: Weigh-ins, particularly the post-exercise weigh-in, are a good opportunity to educate athletes and coaches about the need to consume fluids at a rate no less than equal to the amount of fluids lost by both sweat and urine during prolonged exercise.[1]

When athletes are exposed to hot environments over time, their bodies have the ability to adapt in many ways. This process of physiological adaptation is referred to as heat acclimatization. According to the National Athletic Trainers' Association, the heat acclimatization period for secondary school athletes is the first 2 weeks or 14 days of practice during the preseason.[2] During this period of bodily adjustment, over time, as the body is exposed to a hot and/or humid environment, many important changes take place that, in theory, decrease an athlete's risk of heat illness. Some of these heat acclimatization changes include an increase in sweat rate, a more uniform bodily sweat pattern, and improved conservation of sodium or salt during shorter bouts of exercise. As a result, weigh-ins are going to be affected during this acclimatization process, and educating athletes about these changes will assist them in adjusting their fluid intake during exercise.

A common question often asked is "How long do athletes need to be weighed in and weighed out to properly monitor them in a hot environment?" It's a very good

Table 33-1

Heat Illness Watchlist Chart

Body Weight (lb)	1% Lost (lb)	2% Lost (lb)	3% Lost (lb)	4% Lost (lb)
120	118	117	116	115
125	123	122	121	120
130	128	127	126	124
135	133	132	130	129
140	138	137	135	134
145	143	142	140	139
150	148	147	145	144
155	153	151	150	148
160	158	156	155	153
165	163	161	160	158
170	168	166	164	163
175	173	171	169	168
180	178	176	174	172
185	183	181	179	177
190	188	186	184	182
195	193	191	189	187
200	198	196	194	192
205	202	200	198	196
210	207	205	203	201
215	212	210	208	206
220	217	215	213	211
225	222	220	218	216
230	227	225	223	220
235	232	230	227	225
240	237	235	232	230
245	242	240	237	235
250	247	245	242	240
255	252	249	247	244
260	257	254	252	249
265	262	259	257	254
270	267	264	261	259

(continued)

Table 33-1 (continued)
Heat Illness Watchlist Chart

Body Weight (lb)	1% Lost (lb)	2% Lost (lb)	3% Lost (lb)	4% Lost (lb)
275	272	269	266	264
280	277	274	271	268
285	282	279	276	273
290	287	284	281	278
295	292	289	286	283
300	297	294	291	288

question. The best answer is to continue pre- and post-workout and game weigh-ins for the first 4 weeks of all team-organized workouts. As the athletes become more heat acclimatized during the first few weeks of practice, their increased sweat rates will increase their fluid needs. Continuing the weigh-ins will ensure that the athletes are adequately replacing lost fluids during this time. As for football players, because of the intensity and duration of the workouts and games, it is good practice to continue with this plan up to and including the third regular-season game. The involvement of football equipment may increase sweat rate and greatly increases the concern for heat illness; therefore, more aggressive steps should be taken to educate, hydrate, and monitor athletes involved with this sport.[3]

It's very important to note, as with all medical plans, that there are always exceptions to the rule. According to the Korey Stringer Institute,[4] the following list of factors will increase an athlete's potential risk for heat illness:

- Poor fitness/obesity
- Insufficient fluid consumption
- Fever
- Gastrointestinal dysfunction
- Intense and prolonged exercise in an elevated hot and humid environment

This list serves as a great example of conditions that merit an athlete to continue to be weighed before and after activity. It would be wise to continue to do so until the condition is completely eliminated, and a physician agrees with discontinuing the need to monitor the athlete's weight.

Weighing an athlete immediately before and after an activity is a simple step to help keep your athletes safe. As previously mentioned, Table 33-1 can serve as an easy guide to help in determining the percentage of body mass lost during a given exercise bout. It takes little effort by all parties to accomplish this, so there should be little concern to quickly discontinuing this step if the athletes are at any risk. Athletes should be educated on how to replace fluids lost during exercise before the next practice, training session, or competition. Any individual who has lost > 2% of his or her body mass may need to be held out from the next exercise bout unless euhydration can be confirmed with urine specific gravity or another valid hydration measure.

References

1. Casa DJ, et al. National Athletic Trainers' Association position statement: exertional heat illnesses. *J Athl Train*. 2015;50.
2. Casa DJ, Csillan D, Armstrong LE, et al. National Athletic Trainers' Association consensus statement: pre-season practice guidelines for high school athletics. *J Athl Train*. 2009;44(3):332-333.
3. Kerr ZY, Casa DJ, Marshall SW, Comstock RD. Epidemiology of exertional heat illness among U.S. high school athletes. *Am J Prev Med*. 2013;44(1):8-14.
4. Korey Stringer Institute. http://ksi.uconn.edu/emergency-conditions/heat-illnesses/exertional-heat-stroke/. Accessed March 11, 2014.

Is It Possible for an Athlete to Become Overhydrated, and Does This Help or Hinder the Athlete?

Dawn M. Emerson, MS, ATC

Overhydration, or hyperhydration, occurs when an individual exceeds a normal (euhydrated) state of fluid balance. An individual may hyperhydrate prior to activity to ensure hydration at the start of exercise or to counteract fluid loss during exercise. For example, hyperhydration may benefit a runner who continuously experiences symptoms of dehydration during a 1-hour run. The runner knows his or her sweat rate is 1.5 L/h and tries to consume enough fluid to match sweat rate. However, the runner experiences gastrointestinal discomfort because of the large volume of fluid needed or does not have access to fluids during the run. The runner may choose to hyperhydrate before running to counteract the dehydration during exercise. There are a variety of hyperhydration methods, each with unique benefits and potential side effects. Common methods include increased water intake, glycerol supplementation, carbohydrate-electrolyte beverage consumption or sodium supplementation, and intravenous (IV) fluid injection.

Theoretically, excessive water consumption would hyperhydrate an individual. However, fluid balance is closely regulated by the kidneys. Rapid water intake

Lopez RM, ed. *Quick Questions in Heat-Related Illness and Hydration: Expert Advice in Sports Medicine* (pp 183-187).
© 2015 Taylor & Francis Group.

increases blood pressure and plasma volume. In an effort to maintain homeostasis and rid excess water, hormonal responses in conjunction with the kidneys cause diuresis (increased urine output). Therefore, a rapid ingestion of water will not necessarily allow someone to achieve hyperhydration. To avoid these hormonal responses, a metered approach may be considered, where the individual consumes a standard amount of fluid over time (eg, 100 mL every 15 min for 1 h). This approach allows the body time to absorb the water and establish a hyperhydrated state.

Water intake alone can effectively establish euhydration prior to exercise, but extreme caution should be used if attempting hyperhydration. Whether through metered or rapid intake, water hyperhydration increases the risk for developing hyponatremia. Considered "dilutional hyponatremia," excessive water intake overloads the kidneys' ability to excrete fluids and maintain electrolyte balance. Blood sodium levels become dangerously diluted, and this condition is potentially fatal. A metered approach may decrease hyponatremia risk by allowing self-monitoring of hydration status through urination frequency, urine volume, and/or urine color.

Glycerol is a clear, odorless, sweet-tasting liquid easily metabolized by the body for glycolysis or gluconeogenesis.[1] Glycerol is an effective hyperhydrating agent because of the gradient created between the body's fluid compartments. By increasing solute concentration, fluids flow from outside the compartment (low concentration) to inside the compartment (high concentration). Glycerol also works on the kidneys by promoting fluid reabsorption.[1] Thus, plasma volume increases and hydration is maintained. While it has been inferred that increasing fluid retention during exercise will decrease cardiovascular strain and improve thermoregulation, studies on the exact benefits on core temperature, cardiac function, and performance measures are conflicting. Improvements in these measures are likely secondary to maintaining euhydration. Compared with water, glycerol is considered to be more beneficial in delaying dehydration during exercise.[2] On the other hand, during heat stress it appears that water hyperhydration is as effective as glycerol in maintaining performance and thermoregulation in terms of exercise time, core temperature, and cardiovascular measures.[3]

To be used as a hyperhydrating agent, glycerol must be consumed at low doses, approximately 5 g/100 mL of fluid. At higher doses, 20 to 80 g/100 mL of fluid, glycerol acts as a dehydrating agent.[1] The suggested glycerol hyperhydration protocol is 1.2 g/kg body weight in 26 mL/kg body weight of fluid (water or carbohydrate-electrolyte beverage) over a 60-minute period.[4] Glycerol ingestion is usually well tolerated. However, side effects such as nausea, gastrointestinal distress, headaches, and light-headedness may occur from either glycerol or the large volumes of fluid consumed with it. Individuals with kidney, liver, or cardiovascular disease should not use glycerol supplementation because of the effects on fluid balance.[4]

Last, individuals subject to drug testing by either international or national antidoping agencies or the National Collegiate Athletic Association should avoid glycerol hyperhydration. Glycerol is banned by these agencies because of its effect as a "plasma expander" or as a masking agent. Glycerol is commonly found in foods, and normal consumption of those foods will not result in a positive drug test.

Carbohydrate-electrolyte beverages, or sports drinks, may also be used on their own for hyperhydration. Of the electrolytes present in carbohydrate-electrolyte beverages, sodium is the most effective at promoting fluid retention. Sodium is a cation and, similar to glycerol, exerts an osmotic effect. Where sodium is present, water will follow. Increases in sodium concentration create an osmotic effect that promotes fluid reabsorption through the kidneys and stimulates fluid regulatory hormones to prevent fluid loss. It is unclear how long sodium hyperhydration effects last, but sodium offers additional benefits that water and glycerol alone do not. Sodium hyperhydration can decrease urine production, increase or maintain blood sodium during exercise, and promote fluid intake by stimulating thirst.

Although concentrations vary, most sports drinks contain the recommended sodium content (50 to 100 mmol/L) to promote hydration. On the contrary, some electrolyte supplements contain no sodium; therefore, individuals considering a supplement should check the sodium content. Combining sports drinks and glycerol has been hypothesized to further enhance hyperhydrating effects by increasing the absorption of glycerol while also gaining the benefits of sodium supplementation. Conclusions about whether there is a benefit in humans cannot be made at this time because research in this area is primarily in animal models.

There are some risks associated with sodium/electrolyte hyperhydration. High sodium concentrations make some beverages unpalatable, causing the individual to be less likely to drink the fluid. Excessive sodium, especially with salt tablets, may cause nausea, vomiting, or gastrointestinal distress. Last, individuals with high blood pressure or cardiovascular disease, especially if instructed to reduce dietary sodium, should not use sodium hyperhydration.

A less practical hyperhydration method is IV fluid injection. Collegiate and professional athletes may use IV fluid injection pre-exercise for a variety of reasons, including hyperhydration. However, the limited research available has failed to show improvement in physiological or perceptual measures with IV hyperhydration versus oral fluid intake.[5] The benefit of hyperhydration through normal saline IV fluid is the direct increase in plasma volume and subsequent delay in dehydration during activity, similar to glycerol and sodium. Obvious risks of using IV fluid are those associated with the injection. Use of IV fluids as a prophylactic may also violate the "no needles" policies enforced by many sports' governing bodies. As with excessive oral water ingestion, the use of hypotonic saline poses the risk of developing hyponatremia.

Table 34-1

Advantages and Disadvantages of Pre-Exercise Hyperhydration Techniques

Hyperhydration Method	Advantage	Disadvantage
Oral water ingestion	Increases plasma volume	Hyponatremia risk Least effective method of delaying dehydration during exercise Increases urine output
Glycerol supplement	Increases plasma volume Increases kidney fluid reabsorption more effectively than water Decreases urine output	Banned by World Anti-Doping Agency and National Collegiate Athletic Association Contraindicated in kidney, liver, or cardiovascular disease May cause gastrointestinal distress, headaches, or lightheadedness
Carbohydrate-electrolyte beverage (sodium)	Increases plasma volume Increases kidney fluid reabsorption Stimulates hormones to prevent fluid loss Increases thirst to promote fluid intake Decreases urine output Maintains plasma sodium concentration	Contraindicated in hypertension and other cardiovascular disease May cause gastrointestinal distress High sodium content may be difficult to palate
IV fluid injection	Directly increases plasma volume	Invasive May violate "no needle policy" As effective as oral water ingestion

An individual's hydration protocol should include pre-exercise considerations, and may include hyperhydration techniques if warranted. Despite the possible benefits of hyperhydration, there are a number of serious risks to consider before attempting these techniques (Table 34-1). Consider the previous example of the runner. Despite knowing his or her sweat rate and attempting to consume an equal volume of fluid, the runner consistently experiences dehydration during exercise. Using water alone may decrease the runner's sodium and is not as effective as glycerol and sodium at delaying dehydration during exercise. Glycerol and sodium will establish pre-exercise hyperhydration and delay dehydration during exercise, but each brings unique disadvantages (see Table 34-1). It appears that IV fluid injection is as effective at delaying dehydration as water consumption, but on average IV fluid injection is an impractical method. It is important to note that regardless of the technique, hyperhydration pre-exercise does not negate the importance of consuming fluids (water, sports drinks, etc) during activity to maintain hydration.

References

1. Nelson JL, Robergs RA. Exploring the potential ergogenic effects of glycerol hyperhydration. *Sports Med.* 2007;37(11):981-1000.
2. O'Brien CP, Fruend BJ, Young AJ, Sawka MN. Glycerol hyperhydration: physiological responses during cold-air exposure. *J Appl Physiol.* 2005;99:7.
3. Marino FE, Kay D, Cannon J. Glycerol hyperhydration fails to improve endurance performance and thermoregulation in humans in a warm humid environment. *Pflugers Arch.* 2003;446(4):455-462.
4. van Rosendal SP, Osborne MA, Fassett RG, Coombes JS. Guidelines for glycerol use in hyperhydration and rehydration associated with exercise. *Sports Med.* 2010;40(2):113-139.
5. Hostler D, Gallagher M, Jr., Goss FL, et al. The effect of hyperhydration on physiological and perceived strain during treadmill exercise in personal protective equipment. *Eur J Appl Physiol.* 2009;105(4):607-613.

WHAT IS HYPONATREMIA, AND HOW CAN IT BE PREVENTED, DIAGNOSED, AND TREATED?

Dawn M. Emerson, MS, ATC

Etiology

Sodium is imperative to the proper function of certain body systems. Consequently, sodium balance is tightly regulated, and small changes below normal can cause severe side effects. Hyponatremia is defined as plasma sodium concentration less than 135 mEq/L.[1] Exertional hyponatremia occurs when sodium is depleted during physical activity. A number of factors play into the development of exertional hyponatremia, which typically occurs in individuals who participate in long duration, endurance-type exercise lasting longer than 3.5 hours (eg, marathons, triathlons, ultra-distance events). Exertional hyponatremia is not just a concern for endurance sports; it has been observed in hikers, military personnel, and some team sport athletes. Regardless of the sport/activity, it is important for medical personnel and physically active individuals to be aware of the causes, predisposing factors, signs and symptoms, and treatment of this condition.

Lopez RM, ed. *Quick Questions in Heat-Related Illness and Hydration: Expert Advice in Sports Medicine* (pp 189-194).
© 2015 Taylor & Francis Group.

Proposed causes of hyponatremia include overconsumption of water, inadequate dietary sodium intake, and/or excessive sodium loss through sweat or urine. Consuming hypotonic fluid, such as water, in excess of sweat rate dilutes blood sodium levels. Research has shown that a large number of hyponatremic patients who present after activity have gained weight,[2] indicating hyperhydration. However, some hyponatremic patients will present with weight loss, indicating both dehydration and sodium depletion. Hyponatremia associated with dehydration can be attributed to either inadequate dietary sodium intake and/or excessive sodium loss in sweat and urine. Low dietary sodium can be the result of cutting salt out of the diet for health reasons, such as trying to lower blood pressure, or "salty sweaters" unknowingly not consuming adequate sodium because they are unaware of their sodium needs. It is recommended that the average person consume 1.5 g of dietary sodium, but when someone exercises, he or she loses a large amount of sodium in both sweat and urine. An athlete with a sweat rate of 1 L/h exercising for 4 hours in a moderately hot environment will lose 4 L of fluid through sweat alone. If his or her sweat sodium concentration equaled 1g/L, that would be 4 g of sodium loss through sweat during his or her activity, much higher than the recommended daily sodium intake.

The exact etiology of hyponatremia can vary based on the person and number of predisposing factors. Key factors include activity duration, frequency of fluid consumption, gender, heat acclimatization status, and environment. A number of researchers have identified slow runners, females, and frequent fluid consumption (eg, individuals consuming fluids at every mile or every other mile of a marathon) to be at greater risk for developing hyponatremia.[3,4] Slow runners are likely to drink more fluids throughout activity, potentially stopping at every hydration station, or are less physically fit and unaware of their hydration needs. It is unclear why females have a higher risk, potentially because of their smaller body mass or slower running times. Unacclimatized individuals have higher sweat sodium losses, losing greater amounts of sodium than if they were acclimatized. In addition, fluid needs change based upon the environment. Exercising in a hot, humid environment increases sweat loss as the body attempts to cool itself. Other less understood factors include the use of nonsteroidal anti-inflammatory medications and abnormal secretion of arginine vasopressin, an antidiuretic hormone that causes water retention.

Diagnosis

Symptoms of hyponatremia begin to appear when plasma sodium drops to approximately 130 mEq/L.[4] Mild symptoms include weakness, dizziness, headache, vomiting, nausea, swelling of extremities, and abdominal pain. More severe symptoms are coma, seizure, and altered level of consciousness. If left untreated or misdiagnosed, hyponatremia could result in death. It is imperative for clinicians to be able to differentiate hyponatremia from other conditions with similar symptoms. Symptoms of hyponatremia mimic dehydration, exertional heat illnesses, concussions, and other conditions (Table 35-1). A measurement of plasma sodium is needed to make this distinction from other conditions; however, this measurement is difficult to obtain in most athletic settings. Obtaining a plasma sodium measurement requires expensive equipment and technical training. If a sodium analyzer is not available, clinicians must rely on specific patient history to assess for hyponatremia. For example, if the patient is conscious, inquire about his or her fluid consumption and frequency of urination. A patient who has consumed ample fluid and needs to urinate often will most likely not be suffering from dehydration. Comparing pre- and post-exercise body weight will indicate whether an individual has lost or gained fluid weight. An increase in body weight from pre- to post-exercise is more likely to be associated with overconsumption of fluids. To differentiate between heat illnesses, especially exertional heat stroke, assess the patient's core temperature. An individual experiencing hyponatremia will not likely have a core body temperature greater than 104°F. In a potentially hypoglycemic patient, blood glucose can be measured. Medical personnel should take similar steps with an unconscious individual to differentiate causes of collapse. It is important to note that symptoms of hyponatremia may not occur immediately at the conclusion of an event, potentially presenting hours afterward. Athletes should be educated on signs and symptoms of hyponatremia in order to recognize this potentially dangerous condition and receive appropriate medical care.

Treatment

The goal of hyponatremia treatment is to establish normal plasma sodium levels. Patients with mild symptoms and small changes in plasma sodium levels can be treated with fluid restriction and salty foods. As patients with mild hyponatremia urinate, blood levels should return to normal. This treatment may take a few minutes or several hours, and patients should be monitored until they reach normal plasma sodium levels (135 to 145 mEq/L). If it is not possible to measure plasma sodium levels, patients should be monitored until symptoms have dissipated and be referred to a physician for follow-up. If a patient reports with severe symptoms or begins to deteriorate during treatment, this is a medical emergency and he or she should be referred to the emergency department immediately. Use of a hypertonic (3% to 5%) saline infusion is necessary at this point to establish normal sodium levels. The infusion of *hyper*tonic saline is critical, as *hypo*tonic saline would continue to dilute the plasma sodium concentration and exacerbate the patient's condition.

Table 35-1

Comparison of Hyponatremia Symptoms to Conditions in Differential Diagnoses*

	Signs and Symptoms Similar to Hyponatremia	Signs and Symptoms That Differentiate These From Hyponatremia
Exertional heat stroke	Altered mental status Irrational behavior Seizure Coma Death	Rectal temperature > 104°C Plasma sodium > 135 mEq/L Dehydration Hypotension Hyperventilation
Heat exhaustion	Nausea Vomiting Dizziness Fatigue	Plasma sodium > 135 mEq/L Oliguria Dehydration Hypotension
Dehydration	Headache Nausea Vomiting Dizziness Fatigue	Plasma sodium > 135 mEq/L Oliguria Dehydrated status: urine specific gravity > 1.015 Weight loss from pre-post exercise in excess of fluid intake Infrequent fluid intake during exercise Symptoms do not improve with fluid restriction
Concussion/traumatic brain injury	Loss of consciousness Altered mental status Irrational behavior Headache Disorientation Vomiting Dizziness "Pressure in head" Seizure Coma Death	Plasma sodium > 135 mEq/L Amnesia Decreased motor function Photophobia Phonophobia Abnormal cranial nerve assessment Symptoms do not improve with fluid restriction

(continued)

Table 35-1 (continued)

Comparison of Hyponatremia Symptoms to Conditions in Differential Diagnoses*

	Signs and Symptoms Similar to Hyponatremia	Signs and Symptoms That Differentiate These From Hyponatremia
Hypoglycemia	Loss of consciousness	Plasma sodium > 135 mEq/L
	Altered mental status	Blood glucose < 70 mg/dL
	Irrational behavior	Hyperventilation
	Headache	Tachycardia
	Nausea	Hunger
	Dizziness	
	Fatigue	
	Seizure	
	Coma	
	Death	

* Not every patient will present with the exact signs and symptoms listed for each condition. When mechanism is unknown, it is imperative clinicians be aware of multiple differentials. Clinicians should complete a thorough evaluation, including history and diagnostic tools (core temperature, plasma sodium, concussion assessment, etc) to differentiate conditions.

Prevention

Hyponatremia can be prevented through a number of measures. By using personalized hydration protocols, individuals are more likely to consume the amount of fluids they need to replace their losses during activity. If possible, hydration protocols should include volume of fluid, type of fluid, frequency of fluid consumption, and electrolyte replacement strategies for the days leading up to and throughout activity. Self-monitoring hydration status through weight changes and urine color is a useful tool to limit overhydration. In addition, proper nutrition, including adequate dietary sodium, can ensure that the person begins activity in a sodium-balanced state. Before, during, and/or after activity, individuals are encouraged to consume salty foods (eg, chips, pretzels) with water instead of relying on sports drinks alone to replace sodium. There is little to no research on the numerous products (eg, gels, salt tablets) marketed to the general population as sodium supplements. Individuals who are interested in using these products should do so with caution and consider increasing sodium through food, rather than using unresearched supplementations.

Table 35-2

Key Prevention, Predisposing Factors, Signs and Symptoms, and Treatment of Hyponatremia

Prevention	Predisposing Factors	Signs and Symptoms	Treatment
Personal hydration protocol Self-monitor hydration status Proper nutrition/diet	Low-sodium diet Salty sweaters Fluid consumption > sweat loss Activity ≥ 3 hours Unacclimatized to heat Hot, humid environment	Frequent urination Dilute urine Plasma sodium < 135 mEq/L Swelling of extremities Headache	Restrict fluid Provide salty foods Hypertonic saline

Regardless of the type of physical activity, individuals may be at risk for exertional hyponatremia if they are following an inappropriate hydration protocol and/or inadequate dietary sodium intake. For athletic trainers and other medical personnel, identifying risk factors and educating patients on proper hydration is the best way to prevent hyponatremia. Because hyponatremia may present similar to other life-threatening conditions, it is imperative that medical personnel be able to identify signs and symptoms of hyponatremia and use immediate and appropriate treatment. A summary of key factors in prevention, predisposing factors, signs and symptoms, and treatment of hyponatremia is presented in Table 35-2.

References

1. Speedy DB, Rogers IR, Noakes TD, et al. Exercise-induced hyponatremia in ultradistance triathletes is caused by inappropriate fluid retention. *Clin J Sport Med*. Oct 2000;10(4):272-278.
2. Noakes TD, Sharwood K, Speedy D, et al. Three independent biological mechanisms cause exercise-associated hyponatremia: evidence from 2,135 weighed competitive athletic performances. *Proc Natl Acad Sci U S A*. Dec 20 2005;102(51):18550-18555.
3. Almond CS, Shin AY, Fortescue EB, et al. Hyponatremia among runners in the Boston Marathon. *N Engl J Med*. 2005;352(15):1550-1556.
4. Speedy DB, Noakes TD, Rogers IR, et al. Hyponatremia in ultradistance triathletes. *Med Sci Sports Exerc*. Jun 1999;31(6):809-815.

IS DRINKING A SPORTS DRINK MORE BENEFICIAL TO DRINKING WATER FOR EITHER INCREASED PERFORMANCE OR PREVENTING EXERTIONAL HEAT ILLNESS OR HYPONATREMIA?

J. D. Adams, MS and
Stavros A. Kavouras, PhD, FACSM, FECSS

Water ingestion during exercise, especially in the heat, can improve exercise performance and reduce strain in cardiovascular, muscular, and central nervous systems.[1] Recent data indicate that even the ingestion of a small amount of water can enhance exercise performance in the heat.[2] Additionally, carbohydrate and electrolyte intake can provide an additional performance advantage, especially in prolonged and intense exercise. Although ample scientific evidence exists to support that athletes should consume water, carbohydrates, and electrolytes during exercise, the specific recommendations for optimally applying these principles are not simple. This is because of the varied nature of stresses that athletes encounter during training and competition, as well as the unique regulations of each sport regarding the access and availability of fluid intake during competition.

The term *sports drink* refers to a carbohydrate and electrolytes beverage. The specific aims of sports drinks are to provide fluids, stimulate absorption, reduce physiological stress, and enhance exercise performance. Sports drinks are not to be confused with energy drinks, which contain higher amounts of carbohydrates along with caffeine and other ingredients to improve perceptions and mental

Lopez RM, ed. *Quick Questions in Heat-Related Illness and Hydration: Expert Advice in Sports Medicine* (pp 195-198).

Table 36-1

The Composition of
Various Sports Drinks and Other Beverages

	Carbohydrate (%)	Sodium (mmol/L)	Potassium (mmol/L)	Osmolality (mosm/kg)
Gatorade	6	20	3	360
Powerade	6	23	2	280
Orange juice	10	4	45	660
Cola	11	3	1	700
Bottled water	0	0	0	9
Milk	5	26	37	288

alertness. Although a sports drink may contain a wide variety of nutrients and other substances, it comprises mainly water in addition to other components (ie, sodium and carbohydrates), which could otherwise be obtained from food. Most sports drinks have a carbohydrate content between 4% and 8% (4 to 8 g carbohydrates per 100 mL of drink) and contain small amounts of electrolytes, the main one being sodium. The composition of many commercially available sports drinks can be found in the Table 36-1.[3]

Advantages of Sports Drinks

During intense exercise, muscle and liver carbohydrate stores (glycogen) are the main fuel. However, these energy stores are relatively small and can be depleted within 60 minutes of intense exercise, resulting in fatigue. Even though sports drinks contain a small amount of carbohydrates, they can provide enough energy to prolong exercise and enhance performance.[1]

Drinking plain water can improve performance in endurance exercise, but there are further performance improvements when carbohydrate and electrolytes are added. As stated by the American College of Sports Medicine, "carbohydrate consumption can be beneficial to sustain exercise intensity during high-intensity exercise events of approximately 1 hour or longer, as well as less intense exercise events sustained for longer periods."[4] For people who exercise at a moderate intensity for less than 1 hour, and who do not experience fatigue, water could be the drink of choice. Yet, ingesting carbohydrates during events of this nature will provide no impairment.

It is well documented that during exercise, athletes usually drink less than what they lose via sweating, resulting in dehydration. This phenomenon has been described as involuntary dehydration. For many individuals, sports drinks are the drink of choice because of their taste. The palatability of a beverage is important, as individuals who lose large amounts of sweat are more likely to drink more if the taste of the drink is better. Sports drinks also promote fluid retention because of their sodium content, which leads to lower urinary excretion. The existing evidence indicates that this effect is a result of sodium in the drink.[4]

Also, recent scientific data have investigated the role of sports drinks and mouth rinsing on athletic performance, regardless of the mode of exercise. Whether it is a short intense bout of exercise or prolonged endurance event, mouth rinsing with a carbohydrate drink can improve physiological performance, probably by enhancing motivation via brain activation.

During prolonged endurance events, especially when fluid intake exceeds sweat losses, athletes can develop exercise-associated hyponatremia, which is defined as a blood sodium level below 130 mmol/L and occasionally occurs in American football players, tennis players, ironman triathletes, or ultra-marathoners who drink more water than they sweat. Although drinking water is adequate in most situations, it may not be so when sweat losses and fluid intakes are high.[4] Exercise-associated hyponatremia can be prevented by ingesting electrolyte drinks, rather than water, over long periods of time.[5]

Disadvantages of Sports Drinks

The ingestion of sports drinks during exercise may induce gastrointestinal distress, especially when carbohydrate content is greater than 8% to 10%. Because of this fact, athletes who are predisposed to gastrointestinal problems should attempt to identify a sports drink that does not trigger any discomfort. A lower carbohydrate concentration can also help in avoiding gastrointestinal issues. Moreover, sports drinks have been linked to tooth decay because of the sugar content. Even though the data are not conclusive, it is a good idea for athletes to drink sports drinks only during exercise. Last, even though sports drinks provide less energy than most beverages (~60 kcal versus ~100 kcal for a cola drink per glass), they can still contribute to total energy balance and potentially to body weight regulation. If losing weight is an issue, athletes should consume sports drinks only when necessary.

Conclusion

During exercise, water intake can provide an effective and healthy way to improve performance and avoid heat injuries. During exercise a sports drink can provide an additional advantage by providing energy in the form of carbohydrates and electrolytes. Sports drinks provide an advantage over water when intense exercise is performed for more than 1 hour or when exercise is of lower intensity but lasts for a longer duration.

References

1. Coyle EF. Fluid and fuel intake during exercise. *J Sports Sci.* 2004;22(1):39-55.
2. Arnaoutis G, Kavouras SA, Christaki I, Sidossis LS. Water ingestion improves performance compared with mouth rinse in dehydrated subjects. *Med Sci Sports Exerc.* 2012;44(1):175-179.
3. Shirreffs SM. Hydration in sport and exercise: water, sports drinks and other drinks. *Nutr Bull.* 2009;34(4):374-379.
4. Sawka MN, Burke LM, Eichner ER, Maughan RJ, Montain SJ, Stachenfeld NS. American College of Sports Medicine position stand: exercise and fluid replacement. *Med Sci Sports Exerc.* 2007;39(2):377-390.
5. Anastasiou CA, Kavouras SA, Arnaoutis G, et al. Sodium replacement and plasma sodium drop during exercise in the heat when fluid intake matches fluid loss. *J Athl Train.* 2009;44(2):117-123.

WHAT EFFECT DOES HYDRATION STATUS HAVE ON BODY TEMPERATURE DURING EXERCISE?

Matthew A. Tucker, MA and Matthew S. Ganio, PhD

Fluid balance in the body is the balance between water input (from foods, beverages, and a small amount generated by metabolism) and water output (urine, insensible losses, sweat, and fecal loss). During conditions of physiological stress (ie, exercise), the ability to maintain optimal fluid balance (ie, euhydration) has significant implications with regard to core body temperature regulation (referred to simply as *body temperature* throughout). The body's response to increased body temperature during exercise is to increase skin blood flow and sweating. The ability of these thermoregulatory responses to optimally attenuate increases in body temperature is affected by hydration status. For example, a deficit in fluid balance (ie, dehydration) results in a higher body temperature than if euhydration is maintained. A higher body temperature can negatively affect athletic performance, mood state, and cognitive function and can increase one's risk for heat illness (Figure 37-1). This risk is further exacerbated when extreme environmental conditions place additional stress on thermoregulatory function (ie, hot/dry or hot/humid conditions; temperature $\geq 90°F$, $32°C$). This chapter will focus on and

Lopez RM, ed. *Quick Questions in Heat-Related Illness and Hydration: Expert Advice in Sports Medicine* (pp 199-203).
© 2015 Taylor & Francis Group.

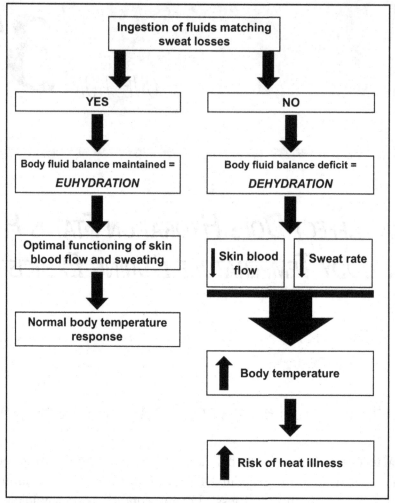

Figure 37-1. Schematic illustrating differences in body temperature response during exercise related to hydration status.

provide the scientific evidence for the relationship between hydration status and body temperature during exercise.

Hydration Status and Its Effect on Thermoregulation

In order to understand how hydration status affects thermoregulation, it is important to understand the basics of thermoregulation. Increased sweat rate and skin blood flow during exercise are the primary thermoregulatory responses to dissipate heat from the body. If sweat rate or blood flow is modulated, thermoregulation, and thus body temperature, will be affected. Indeed, when individuals are dehydrated, skin blood flow and sweat rate are impaired.

Whole-body sweat rate decreases in relation to the level of dehydration.[1] This decrease is partly because a higher body temperature must be reached before sweating will occur, and for the same increase in body temperature there is less sweat produced when an athlete is dehydrated. These impairments are linear, such that the greater the level of dehydration, the greater the level of impairment.[2] Research has shown that sweat rate decreases approximately 50 mL/h for each percent decrease in body weight.[1] Therefore, if an athlete weighing 165 lb loses 3 lb from sweat losses during 1 hour of exercise, he or she has a ~2% body mass loss and will sweat about 100 mL less per hour than if body mass had been maintained while exercising.

Skin blood flow is also affected by hydration status. In one study, during exercise, fluid ingested at a volume to prevent dehydration led to an approximately 20% greater skin blood flow after about 80 minutes of exercise compared with when no fluid was ingested.[3] This implies that dehydration leads to decreased skin blood flow, which hampers the ability of the body to lose heat to the environment. This impaired thermoregulation leads to greater body temperatures.

In summary, when athletes are dehydrated, there is a delay in the onset of sweating, a lowered sweat response, and a decrease in skin blood flow. These impairments are linearly affected with hydration level such that greater dehydration leads to greater impairments. Not surprisingly, this leads to a body temperature increase that is directly related to level of dehydration. For example, an athlete who is dehydrated by -5% body weight will have a higher body temperature than someone who is -3% dehydrated when working at the same workload.

Fluid Intake Before Exercise and Body Temperature Responses

It is important to consider how hydration status prior to exercising may affect body temperature response during exercise. Many sporting activities are not conducive to fluid ingestion during exercise, so it is that much more important that athletes begin the exercise euhydrated. In a classic study, heat-acclimatized males performed 4 prolonged (140 min) treadmill exercise trials in a hot, dry environment starting either euhydrated or dehydrated by 3%, 5%, or 7% of their body weight.[1] Body temperature was lowest in the euhydrated trial and it increased by approximately 0.27°F (0.15°C) for each 1% decrease in body weight. This suggests that hydration status prior to the onset of exercise plays a significant role in the body temperature response.

While previous field studies have examined the relationship between hydration status and body temperature, few have managed to control exercise intensity, a known modulator of body temperature. A recent study was able to control exercise intensity in a field setting.[4] Seventeen heat-acclimatized runners participated in 4 separate trials, each 12 km in length in warm conditions: 2 maximal running races and 2 submaximal runs (maintaining the same pace in the submaximal runs). Half of the trials were conducted when the athletes were euhydrated; half when they were dehydrated. Following the maximal running races, the dehydrated group had a significantly higher body temperature than the euhydrated group. In addition, the euhydrated group completed the trial approximately 2.5 minutes faster than the dehydrated group. Interestingly, in the submaximal trials, body temperature for the dehydrated group was higher both during and after the run. Similar to laboratory studies, body temperature was increased 0.40°F (0.22°C) for every additional 1% of body mass loss. These findings show a clear relationship between baseline hydration status and the degree to which body temperature increases during exercise.

Fluid Intake During Exercise and Body Temperature Responses

Starting exercise while euhydrated is important, but replacing sweat losses during exercise is also important so that dehydration does not occur. A classic study from 1944 was one of the first to demonstrate an association between fluid intake during exercise and body temperature.[5] Subjects were required to walk on a treadmill in hot/dry or hot/humid conditions for up to 6 hours. During exercise, subjects consumed either no water, water at free will (*ad libitum*), or water matching sweat losses. In the cases in which no water was consumed, body temperature steadily increased until the point of exhaustion. In contrast, when water was provided, matching for sweat losses, body temperature increased slightly before reaching a plateau. Consumption of water *ad libitum* also aided in attenuating the increase in body temperature, although body temperature was greater than in the matching sweat loss trial because fluid intake did not match sweat losses. This phenomenon is referred to as "involuntary dehydration," a condition in which humans typically only voluntarily consume about two-thirds the amount of fluids lost in sweat.[5] This shows that during exercise, the rise in body temperature can be attenuated when fluids are consumed in an amount equivalent to sweat losses (ie, preventing a negative fluid balance from occurring). Follow-up studies have confirmed similar findings[3]: body temperature responses are related to the amount of fluid intake during exercise. In other words, if more fluid is ingested during exercise, the body temperature response is lower. However, it is important that individuals do not drink more fluid than is lost through sweating because this can result in a dangerous medical condition called exercise-associated hyponatremia. Exercising individuals should drink enough fluid to replace sweat losses, not more.

Conclusion

There is a large amount of laboratory and field-based data demonstrating a strong relationship between hydration status and body temperature. This relationship holds true when beginning exercise in a euhydrated versus dehydrated state, even if the starting hydration status is maintained throughout exercise with fluid ingestion. If athletes are able to begin physical activity in a euhydrated state and continue to consume fluids during exercise in an amount that prevents a body fluid deficit in excess of approximately 1% (ie, sweating more than is being consumed), skin blood flow and sweating can function optimally. By doing this, athletes will prevent impairment of these responses, keeping their body temperature lower (versus a dehydrated state) and subsequently decrease their risk for developing heat illnesses (see Figure 37-1).

References

1. Sawka MN, Young AJ, Francesconi R, Muza S, Pandolf KB. Thermoregulatory and blood responses during exercise at graded hypohydration levels. *J Appl Physiol.* 1985;59(5):1394-1401.
2. Montain SJ, Latzka WA, Sawka MN. Control of thermoregulatory sweating is altered by hydration level and exercise intensity. *J Appl Physiol.* 1995;79(5):1434-1439.
3. Montain SJ, Coyle E. Influence of graded dehydration on hyperthermia and cardiovascular drift during exercise. *J Appl Physiol.* 1992;73(4):1340-1350.
4. Casa DJ, Stearns RL, Lopez RM, et al. Influence of hydration on physiological function and performance during trail running in the heat. *J Athl Train.* 2010;45(2):147.
5. Pitts G, Johnson R, Consolazio F. Work in the heat as affected by intake of water, salt and glucose. *Am J Physiol.* 1944;142.

Do Supplements (eg, Creatine and Caffeine) Cause Dehydration or Exertional Heat Illness During Activity in Hot Environments?

Candi D. Ashley, PhD

Ergogenic aids such as caffeine and creatine are commonly used to help athletes become bigger, faster, and stronger. Creatine is commonly used to increase performance in anaerobic events, while caffeine is used to enhance aerobic performance. Yet, there is some controversy surrounding the potential negative effects of these ergogenic aids during athletic performance in hot and/or humid environments.

Caffeine is the most widely used drug by athletes and nonathletes alike,[1] and a number of sports drinks and energy drinks are infused with caffeine for that competitive edge. Low to moderate doses of caffeine have been found to enhance endurance performance as a result of increased sympathetic nervous system stimulation and increased fat utilization.[2] Low to moderate doses are 3 to 10 mg/kg, which are equivalent to approximately two to seven 8-ounce cups of brewed coffee for a 70-kg person. Other effects of caffeine include increased sympathetic nervous system stimulation and resting metabolic rate. Caffeine has been shown to increase alertness and reduce feelings of fatigue.[2] However, caffeine

Lopez RM, ed. *Quick Questions in Heat-Related Illness and Hydration: Expert Advice in Sports Medicine* (pp 205-208).
© 2015 Taylor & Francis Group.

ingestion has been purported to lead to dehydration and increased risk of heat illness because of increased diuresis. Because of caffeine's ability to increase resting metabolic rate, which could theoretically increase metabolic heat production, some believe caffeine increases core body temperature, thereby increasing the risk of heat illness.[2]

While caffeine ingestion increases diuresis, it should be noted that several studies have found that caffeine has a diuretic effect equivalent to water, and others have determined that the effects of water and caffeine on diuresis are synergistic.[1-3] As such, there is not sufficient scientific evidence to support restricting caffeine intake to reduce thermal stress. This is because acute diuresis does not necessarily lead to chronic depletion of body water. Scientific studies have found that caffeine ingestion does bring about an increase in urine production, but it has no effect on 24-hour water balance or 24-hour urinary electrolyte balance, or core body temperature; nor does it have an effect on 24-hour sweat electrolyte balance or sweat rate.[2] This is important because most fluid losses during exercise are the result of sweating, and the evaporation of this sweat from the skin is the primary means of heat dissipation during exercise. There is some evidence of increased urinary sodium excretion with caffeine consumption, but generally the Western diet is abundant in sodium and should replace any losses.[2] While caffeine consumed before or after exercise does increase urine output, there appears to be no diuretic effect when caffeine is consumed during exercise. This may be because of a reduction in blood flow to the kidneys, which commonly occurs during exercise, especially during higher intensity exercise.[3] In conclusion, the available research has demonstrated that caffeine does not impair hydration, exacerbate dehydration, or impair thermoregulation.[4] In fact, caffeinated beverages may contribute to hydration similarly to water.

Energy drinks are one of the most popular supplements for young adult athletes as well as nonathletes. They generally contain caffeine in moderate doses, but some energy drinks contain more than 500 mg of caffeine per serving.[4] That's equivalent to five 8-ounce cups of coffee! Because these drinks are not controlled by the US Food and Drug Administration (FDA), they may contain "other herbal blends," including ephedra, that increase the stimulatory effects of caffeine and can lead to insomnia, nervousness, headache, and tachycardia.[4] The danger lies in the actual amounts and ingredients in the herbal blends. In addition, it can increase the risk of hypertension, stroke, cardiovascular events, and exertional heat illness, especially in athletes exercising in hot and humid conditions.[1,4] It is thought that ephedra may stimulate dopamine receptors, causing vasoconstriction and impaired convective heat loss.[1]

Creatine is used by athletes who compete in short-burst, high-intensity activities. Creatine is a chemical that is found in skeletal muscles. It is made by the body and can be obtained in the diet through fish and meats.[1] Creatine supplementation is believed to increase the content of phosphocreatine in the muscle cell.[1] Phosphocreatine is used to rapidly increase ATP production in the skeletal muscle and thus increase high-intensity, short-duration performance (particularly bouts of exercise lasting < 10 seconds).[1] One side effect of creatine ingestion is an increased intracellular water retention in the muscle cells. This is likely the reasoning behind the anecdotal reports of increased muscle cramping and gastrointestinal distress, renal damage, and impairment of thermoregulation with creatine supplementation. However, there is no scientific evidence to support the contention that creatine supplementation impedes heat tolerance or hydration,[1] and researchers agree that moderate creatine usage is safe.[1,5] Despite numerous studies specifically looking to determine creatine supplementation's effect on hydration and thermoregulation, studies have found no increase in core body temperature with creatine supplementation and no impairments to hydration status.[5] In fact, there have been reports of less of a rise in core body temperature during exercise in those who use creatine.[5] This may be because of the osmotic effects of creatine. With the increased uptake of creatine by the muscles, there is also an increased uptake of water into the muscle cells. This results in a decrease in water in the extracellular spaces, making the extracellular fluid hyperosmotic. The extra fluid in the muscle cells will diffuse into the hyperosmotic fluid in the extracellular spaces, enabling greater fluid for sweat production and plasma volume, thus reducing thermal strain.[5] Theoretically, this could be advantageous for athletes exercising in the heat.

All athletes and coaches want to win. Dietary supplements such as caffeine and creatine are easily attainable and may provide that competitive edge. However, caution should be exercised. Because the FDA does not regulate dietary supplements, the exact amounts and ingredients in a supplement are unknown. And while scientific evidence does suggest that moderate doses of most dietary supplements are safe, anecdotal reports of negative health effects are generally blamed on the "more is better" mentality: athletes take more than the "safe" dose or add several "safe" doses together. Caffeine and creatine supplementation can be safe and effective when taken in moderate amounts (Table 38-1).

Table 38-1

Effects of Caffeine and Creatine Supplementation During Exercise

	Caffeine	Creatine
Sources	Coffee, tea, cola, chocolate	Beef, poultry, fish
Ergogenic effects	Increased aerobic performance	Increased anaerobic power
Average safe dose for performance effects	3 to 10 mg/kg of body weight per day	20 to 25 g/day
Effect on body temperature	None	None
Effect on hydration status	Diuretic effect at rest; no effect with exercise	None

References

1. Lopez RM, Casa DJ. The influence of nutritional ergogenic aids on exercise heat tolerance and hydration status. *Clin Sports Med Rep.* 2009;8(4):192-199.
2. Armstrong LE, Casa DJ, Maresh CM, Ganio MM. Caffeine, fluid-electrolyte balance, temperature regulation, and exercise-heat tolerance. *Exer Sport Sci Rev.* 2007;35(3):135-140.
3. DelCoso J, Estevez E, Mora-Rodriguez R. Caffeine during exercise in the heat: thermoregulation and fluid-electrolyte balance. *Med Sci Sports Exer.* 2009;41(1):164-173.
4. Hoffman JR. Caffeine and energy drinks. *Strength Conditioning J.* 2010;32(1):15-20.
5. Lopez RM, Casa DJ, McDermott BP, et al. Does creatine supplementation hinder exercise heat tolerance or hydration status? A systematic review with meta-analyses. *J Athl Train.* 2009;44(2):215-223.

Is It Possible to Be Well Hydrated and Still Experience Exertional Heat Illness?

Evan C. Johnson, PhD and
Stavros A. Kavouras, PhD, FACSM, FECSS

The short answer to this question is yes. However, all sports medicine providers and coaches should understand that exertional heat illness (EHI) is an umbrella term that encompasses a spectrum of negative physiologic responses related to exercise in the heat. These include, in order of increasing severity, exertional heat cramps, heat syncope, exercise heat exhaustion, and exertional heat stroke (EHS).[1] Exertional hyponatremia is sometimes grouped with EHI and has thus been included. Water is related to all of the above ailments. Most are closely related to the body's fluid/electrolyte balance, while EHS is related to the influence of water as a cooling agent. Because exercise in the heat results in sweating (ie, fluid loss), it is obvious that personal hydration status has been identified as a common risk factor among EHI. However, there are several other risk factors that must also be considered. In this response we will focus on the cause of each of these and how hydration status is and is not related.

Exertional heat cramps are a specific type of muscular cramp that occurs during or following substantial exercise (duration and/or intensity) and sweating. The

Lopez RM, ed. *Quick Questions in Heat-Related Illness and Hydration: Expert Advice in Sports Medicine* (pp 209-213).

common consensus is that the cramping is related to intense muscular contractions combined with electrolyte imbalance caused by sweating.[2] Along with water, sweat also contains electrolytes such as sodium. Thus, if an individual is matching sweat losses by consuming a low-electrolyte beverage, such as water, he or she may be diluting his or her electrolyte concentrations and placing him- or herself at greater risk for cramping. Thus, adequate hydration with water only in some circumstances may predispose an individual to exertional heat cramps. Overall, the best route to take for prevention is to ensure acclimatization to the competition environment, and, if prone to cramping, by drinking fluids with additional salt before, during, and after competition.

Heat syncope is defined as a fainting episode that occurs in an individual with a nonhyperthermic core temperature (ie, < 40°C) who has been exercising in the heat. The cause is insufficient blood flow to the brain and a drop in blood pressure. During exercise in the heat, blood is shunted to the skin's surface from the deep musculature in order to aid in removal of heat from the body. This stress, combined with the blood demand from working muscles, can reduce the amount of blood that returns to the heart. Dehydration can exacerbate this form of EHI because of a reduced total blood volume that further stretches the body's resources for oxygen delivery and heat dissipation. However, heat syncope typically occurs in unacclimatized individuals independently of hydration status when they stand still following prolonged exertion and blood pools in the legs.[3]

Exertional heat exhaustion refers to the fatigue, weakness, and the failure to continue exercise while in a hot environment that occurs because of cardiovascular insufficiency. The cardiovascular insufficiency is typically a result of reduced blood volume either from inadequate fluid or sodium replacement.[3] Obviously, heat exhaustion that results from water depletion can be prevented by adequate hydration. However, heat exhaustion that results from salt depletion typically occurs over consecutive days of exercise in the heat, where more sodium is lost from sweating than is consumed. Reduced total body sodium yields reduced blood volume because, without sodium, water consumed during and following exercise cannot be retained. Therefore, in cases of heat exhaustion from sodium and/or electrolyte depletion an athlete can experience heat exhaustion independently of their efforts to hydrate with low-electrolyte beverages, such as water.

The previous ailments result from fluid/electrolyte imbalance, which is stimulated by the high rates of water turnover that occur during exercise. EHS, on the other hand, is the result of excess stored body heat. Body water is integral to removal of heat from the body because it is the principal component of blood, which directs metabolic heat created by exercising muscles to the skin surface, and also sweat, which allows the heat brought to the surface to be exchanged with the environment by evaporation. However, when body water is low from inadequate pre-event hydration or prolonged sweating without replacement, blood volume shrinks, limiting the heat dissipation mechanism. This can result in up to 0.25°C greater gain in core temperature for each 1% of body mass lost.[4] Thus, mechanistically, water plays a big role in storage of excess body heat above the body's threshold of approximately 40°C. However, lack of sufficient water is not the only method by which normal thermoregulation can be impaired. Through retrospective analysis, the following risk factors have been identified as being common to EHS: being male, some medications and sports supplements (particularly those that increase metabolic rate or contain stimulants), increased age, nonporous clothing (ie, hazardous material suits, football uniform), current illness, poor cardiovascular fitness, inadequate acclimation, or sleep deprivation (Table 39-1).[5] High exercise intensity combined with inadequate rest intervals can also lead to excessive heat storage. Externally, the most significant risk factor to consider is environmental temperature and, more importantly, humidity. Regardless of hydration status, if it is exceedingly hot and humid outside, normal thermoregulation will be substantially reduced, meaning that heat storage will occur at a much faster rate.[2]

Although some sources do not include exertional hyponatremia among the heat illness spectrum, it is most often related to excessive water intake during exercise in the heat. This is a rare response to overdrinking water, in which blood sodium becomes diluted because under normal circumstances a decrease of blood sodium leads to major diuresis to maintain fluid balance. Regardless, it is likely that individuals who attain hyponatremic status began exercise in either a euhydrated or a hyperhydrated state. Furthermore, the worst treatment for an individual with hyponatremia is forced fluid intake with low-electrolyte content beverages, as this will only further dilute the blood. Thus, in order to reduce risk of hyponatremia, a "well hydrated" individual needs to avoid overdrinking.

As we see here, water is directly related to the etiology of the full range of EHI, whether due to improper water/electrolyte balance, or to water's role in body heat dissipation. It is easy to see why individuals may assume (as a result of water loss from sweating) that adequate hydration before, during, and after exercise in the heat could prevent EHI. However, the take-home message here is that just because water is related to the ailment does not mean that drinking enough to limit body mass loss will exclude EHI possibility. This myth is potentially hazardous because the belief that consuming adequate water eliminates risk of EHI could lead to improper precautions being followed (ie, limiting exercise intensity in very hot environments or when sick). Additionally, the belief that poor hydration is the root cause of heat illness may be a contributing factor to some individuals' propensity to overdrink prior to or during exercise in the heat. In order for an individual to be considered "well hydrated," he or she should consume neither too little nor too much water. Coaches and athletes must realize the signs and symptoms of EHI,

Table 39-1

Various Predisposing Factors or Warning Signals of Exertional Heat Stroke Patients[5]

Predisposing Factor or Warning Signal	Number of Prior Heat Stroke Patients Who Acknowledged This Factor (N=10)*
Sleep loss	7
Generalized fatigue	6
A warning sign of impending illness	6
A long exercise bout or workout	5
A long heat exposure (eg, mowing grass, physical training)	5
A heat wave	4
Reduced sweat secretion	3
Fever or disease	3
Dizzy, lightheaded	2
Dehydration	1
Taking medication (ie, antihistamine)	1
Excessive use of alcohol	1
Excessive use of caffeine	1
Consumption of a low salt diet	1
Previous heat illness	1
Sunburn or skin rash	1
Immunization or inoculation	0
Use of diuretics	0
Previous difficulty with exercise in the heat	0
Diarrhea or vomiting	0

* During the 5 days prior to heat stroke episode.
Reprinted with permission from Armstrong LE, De Luca JP, Hubbard RW. Time course of recovery and heat acclimation ability of prior exertional heatstroke patients. *Med Sci Sports Exer.* 1990;22(1):36-48.

particularly EHS, and discontinue exercise when risk is apparent. Continuing exercise in the face of EHS while relying on fluid consumption to mitigate risk could be catastrophic. Overall, there is no doubt that proper hydration is important to exercise in the heat; however, it does not eliminate risk of EHI.

References

1. Armstrong LE. *Exertional Heat Illness.* Champaign, IL: Human Kinetics; 2003.
2. Bergeron MF. Reducing sports heat illness risk. *Pediatr Rev.* 2013;34(2013):270-279.
3. Casa DJ, et al. National Athletic Trainers' Association position statement: exertional heat illnesses. *J Athl Train.* 2015;50.
4. Sawka MN, Montain SJ, Latzka WA. Hydration effects on thermoregulation and performance in the heat. *Comp Biochem Physiol A Mol Integr Physiol.* 2001;128(4):679-690.
5. Armstrong LE, De Luca JP, Hubbard RW. Time course of recovery and heat acclimation ability of prior exertional heatstroke patients. *Med Sci Sports Exer.* 1990;22(1):36-48.

FINANCIAL DISCLOSURES

J. D. Adams has no financial or proprietary interest in the materials presented herein.

William M. Adams has no financial or proprietary interest in the materials presented herein.

Dr. Candi D. Ashley has no financial or proprietary interest in the materials presented herein.

Dr. Joseph S. Atkin has no financial or proprietary interest in the materials presented herein.

Luke N. Belval has no financial or proprietary interest in the materials presented herein.

Michele C. Benz has no financial or proprietary interest in the materials presented herein.

Dr. Douglas J. Casa has no financial or proprietary interest in the materials presented herein.

Dr. Michelle A. Cleary has no financial or proprietary interest in the materials presented herein.

Dr. Earl R. "Bud" Cooper has no financial or proprietary interest in the materials presented herein.

Dr. Eric E. Coris has no financial or proprietary interest in the materials presented herein.

Dr. Julie K. DeMartini has no financial or proprietary interest in the materials presented herein.

Deanna M. Dempsey has no financial or proprietary interest in the materials presented herein.

Dr. Lindsey E. Eberman has no financial or proprietary interest in the materials presented herein.

Dawn M. Emerson has no financial or proprietary interest in the materials presented herein.

Dr. Matthew S. Ganio has no financial or proprietary interest in the materials presented herein.

Yuri Hosokawa has no financial or proprietary interest in the materials presented herein.

Dr. Robert A. Huggins has not disclosed any relevant financial relationships.

Dr. Evan C. Johnson has no financial or proprietary interest in the materials presented herein.

Dr. Stavros A. Kavouras has no financial or proprietary interest in the materials presented herein.

Dr. Rebecca M. Lopez has no financial or proprietary interest in the materials presented herein.

Dr. Brendon P. McDermott receives research support from PreventaMed, Inc.

Nicole E. Moyen has no financial or proprietary interest in the materials presented herein.

Dr. Francis G. O'Connor has no financial or proprietary interest in the materials presented herein.

Dr. Robert C. Oh has no financial or proprietary interest in the materials presented herein.

Dr. Nicholas D. Peterkin has no financial or proprietary interest in the materials presented herein.

J. Luke Pryor has no financial or proprietary interest in the materials presented herein.

Riana R. Pryor has no financial or proprietary interest in the materials presented herein.

Mike D. Ryan has no financial or proprietary interest in the materials presented herein.

Dr. Rebecca L. Stearns has no financial or proprietary interest in the materials presented herein.

Matthew A. Tucker has no financial or proprietary interest in the materials presented herein.

Lesley W. Vandermark has no financial or proprietary interest in the materials presented herein.

INDEX

Printed in the United States
by Baker & Taylor Publisher Services